Body of
Knowledge

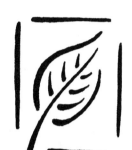

The Beauty Professional's Guide to Career Consciousness Through Self-Care

Mary Beth Janssen

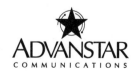
ADVANSTAR
COMMUNICATIONS

Printed in the United States of America

10 9 8 7 6 5 4 3 2 1

ISBN 0-929870-60-3
Library of Congress Control Number 2001087617

Published by Advanstar Communications Inc.

Advanstar Communications is a worldwide business information company that publishes magazines, directories, and books, produces expositions and conferences, provides a wide range of marketing services, and maintains numerous Websites.

Mary Beth Janssen and Advanstar Communications wish to thank The Chopra Center for Well Being for permission to use the Mind Body Questionnaire developed by David Simon, M.D., Medical Director and Co-Founder of The Chopra Center for Well Being. The questionnaire appears on page 59.

For additional information on any Advanstar product or for a complete catalog of published books, please write to: Advanstar Customer Service, 131 West 1st Street, Duluth, Minnesota, 55802 USA; or visit www.advanstar.com.

To purchase additional copies of *Body of Knowledge*, please call 1-800-598-6008; outside the U.S. call 218-723-9180. Order on-line at www.advanstarbooks.com/bok.

ATTENTION TEACHERS, SEMINAR LEADERS, ORGANIZATIONS, COLLEGES AND UNIVERSITIES: Quantity discounts are available on bulk purchases of this book for educational purposes. For more information, please call 1-800-598-6008 or outside the U.S. at 218-723-9180.

Publisher/Product Manager: Danell M. Durica
Editor: Donna Shryer, Chicago IL
Interior Design: Lachina Publishing Services, Inc., Cleveland, OH
Cover Design: Epic Software Group, The Woodlands, TX
Illustrator: Alison Kolesar, Williamstown, MA

Contents

Introduction
Working from the Heart   1
Everyone has the intuitive intelligence to achieve career
consciousness through self-awareness. Everyone.

Chapter One
Behold the Beauty Within   5
Positively affirm your own beauty and you ignite a spark of energy
that radiates outward. This becomes a gift to yourself as well as to
all others you meet.

Chapter Two
Taking Care of the Caregiver   27
Tend to your own self-care first in order to optimize interaction
with all other people—clients included.

Chapter Three
Beauty in Mind, Body, and Spirit   41
Discover new ways and places to find beauty and, in the process,
learn to see beauty on a profoundly deeper level.

Chapter Four
Life's Great Balancing Act   68
Learn how to identify, cope with, and alleviate stress—one of the
most important things you can do for yourself.

Chapter Five
Mindfulness in Motion   96
Create harmony between body, mind, and spirit through joyful
physical activity, be it daily repetitive motions or organized exercise.

Chapter Six
Nourishing Wisdom   134
Nourish your body and soul with food.

Chapter Seven
Sensory Awareness   167
Experience your inner and outer world by appreciating and
protecting your five senses.

Chapter Eight
A Conclusion That Marks the Beginning   207
Reexamining your definition of holistic beauty care.

Epilogue
In Continuation—The World of Holistic Beauty Care   215
You belong to a career-minded community where body, mind,
soul, actions, services, products, and environment all come
together in divine energy.

Resources   225

Bibliography and Recommended Reading   234

Index   241

Dedicated to Xenon:

In Your light I learn how to love.
In your beauty, how to make poems.
You dance inside my chest,
where no one sees you,
But sometimes I do,
and that sight becomes this art.

—*Rumi*

About the Author

MARY BETH JANSSEN, internationally acclaimed educator, author, and beauty and wellness professional, is one of the most well-known women in the beauty profession today.

Her 25+ years of expertise has made her a sought-after talent for magazine editorial, television shows, and commercials. She is a regular speaker at prestigious industry events. She has produced and directed numerous published works in print as well as video and film for major companies in the beauty industry. She's authored several books including *Naturally Healthy Hair* (Storey Publishing 1999) and *Radiant Beauty: Your Healthy and Organic Guide to Total Well-Being* (Rodale Press, 2001).

Based in Chicago, Ms. Janssen currently oversees and directs all activities at The Janssen Source, Inc. As a wellness consultant to the professional beauty industry, Mary Beth brings a message of beauty and wellness integration into the salon and spa environment—a message that is quite specific and transformative for the cosmetologist who Mary Beth likens to a "caregiver."

Ms. Janssen was personally certified by Deepak Chopra, M.D., and David Simon, M.D., as a mindbody health educator for Infinite Possibilities Knowledge, the education arm of Deepak's organization, the Chopra Center for Well-Being. She is also a certified herbalist, aromatherapist, massage therapist, and yoga teacher.

Acknowledgments

I would like to thank my beloved husband, James, the light of my life, my reality check and best critic, and a joy in every part of my world.

I also want to deeply thank my wonderful family, especially my parents, Hubert and Nelly. Your compassion and love have no bounds.

For their help in incubating and supporting who I am and what my work is about, I would like to express my heartfelt thanks and love to the following people and communities—confidantes, friends, guides, mentors, fellow path seekers:

- Donna Shryer for your sensitive, intuitive, and inspired editorial guidance. Without you, this book would not have become a reality.
- Danell Durica, Ted Mathews, and the folks at Advanstar Publishing for their belief in this project, and bringing it to fruition. This includes Lachina Publishing Services, Inc., and Robbin McClain, Hazel Van Landingham, David Wahl, and the many others at Advanstar for your continuing enthusiasm, trust, and support of my message.
- Deepak Chopra, Dr. David Simon, and Roger Gabriel for your expansive and awe-inspiring contributions toward raising universal consciousness. And to my loving "family" at The Chopra Center, especially Nan Johnson, Patty Johnson, Jude Hedlund, and Leanne Backer.
- Leo Passage for your brilliant and nurturing guidance in creating an environment at Pivot Point International where I absolutely thrived. And to all my dear friends, past and present, at Pivot Point International, especially Judy Rambert, Jan Laan, Robert Passage, and Corinne Passage.
- Vi Nelson for your enduring wit, wisdom, inimitable style, and friendship.

- David Raccuglia for your friendship, as well as our shared devotion to those principles that I cherish in the realm of deep ecology and organic living, serenity, and wellness.
- Vidal Sassoon and Horst Rechelbacher for the pure and holistic inspiration you have both shared with the beauty community.
- All my dear friends within the mop family—the "organic web," if you will—including those at the companies' nucleus, the beauty professionals that I've visited in mop salons and spas, and the many devoted distributors and salon consultants that I've had the opportunity to commune with.
- Mary Atherton and Vicki Wurdinger, friends and truly the god-mothers of my writing career.
- My dear friends and mentors alike, Dwight Miller, Carlos Valenzuela, Jeanne Braa, Vivienne Mackinder, Luis Alvarez, Ruth Roche, Teri Donnelly, Gordon Miller, and Jody Byrne.
- Mary Rector, Jackie Summers, and all my friends at Behind the Chair.
- Paul Dykstra, Bob Seidl, Nancy Flinn, Greg and Joanne Starkman, Pamela Lappies, Janice McCafferty, my friends at Katherine-Frank Creative and at ISO—all a part of my evolution.
- My friends at *Modern Salon* and *American Salon Magazines, Salon News, Day Spa Magazine*, NCA, CC—Chicago Cosmetologists, and The Salon Association.
- My dear "girl" friends, what beautiful souls you are! Bea Sochor, Susan Macleary, Leslie Pace, Lynn Maestro, and Ellen Folan.

My love and thanks to all the beauty professionals who have touched my life and to my students—past, present, and future. You are all part of the beautiful tapestry of my life. I do believe in the Latin aphorism—"by learning, you will teach, and by teaching you will learn." I'm inspired and blessed by you all.

And to my dear friend Xenon, I look forward to seeing you on the other side. Namaste'.

A Note to the Reader

The information in this book is not intended as a substitute for the advice of physicians or other qualified health professionals. It is not intended to be prescriptive with reference to any specific ailment or condition or to the general health of the reader but, rather, descriptive of one approach to fostering health and wellness. The reader is advised to consult with his or her physician before undertaking any of the practices contained in this book. The reader should also continue to consult regularly with his or her physician in matters relating to his or her health, particularly in respect to any symptoms that may require diagnosis or medical treatment. Neither the author nor the publisher shall be liable or responsible for any loss, injury, or damage allegedly arising from the use of any information contained in this book.

Working from the Heart

> **Let** the beauty we love
> be what we do.
> *Rumi*

The beauty profession is truly a medium through which we express our vitality, our life-force energy, our absolute uniqueness. For most of us—your author included—understanding and appreciating these truths requires a lifelong spiritual journey. It is and will remain forever an enlightening pilgrimage that teaches us to respect our sense of self, revere our deepest intuitive intelligence, and honor our chosen livelihood.

Every one of us has this intuitive intelligence within—an innate sense that tells us how to achieve self-awareness and career consciousness. This insight constitutes an awakening of our spirituality. When you listen to the spirit within, you are working from the heart and connecting to the most vital part of your individual wisdom. Suddenly you are more able to nurture relationships, relieve anxiety, lessen stress, clear emotional and creative blocks, and accelerate the healing process.

While these achievements are deeply healing for you, they also create awesome residual effects, healthfully influencing every person who enters your personal and professional world. As you learn to work from the heart, simplify your life, tap into your spiritual energy, and optimize nutritional intake as well as movement, you will find that your own healthy state enables you to better provide transformative, beautifying, feel-good services to clients.

1

> *If the doors of perception were cleansed, everything would appear to man as it is—infinite.*
>
> *William Blake*

The question "How may I serve you?" shifts from a routine courtesy to a genuine query. The self-centered and self-absorbed message: "I'll help you, but only if there's something in it for me!" is not acceptable. Instead, this question will represent an unselfish, caring question stated from the heart.

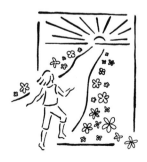

The body of knowledge in this book is meant to challenge you as a beauty professional, prompting you to inventory facets of your personal life, change any aspects that feel uncomfortable, and thus achieve a beautiful, balanced wholeness. This wholeness will absolutely permit you to rekindle or maintain a passion for the beauty profession, and consequently empower you to serve clients in a healthful, creative, and loving way.

To accomplish all this, we'll examine concepts and techniques such as positive affirmation, creative visualization, meditation, bodywork, Pranayama (breathing practices), yoga, and many other enlightening practices. We'll investigate ways to heighten creativity, intuition, and resiliency, as well as our listening powers. Together we will contemplate methods to seamlessly integrate beauty and wellness into all facets of personal life as well as the professional work experience and environment. Because our chosen profession is surprisingly physical (think standing on your feet *all* day), we'll address how to maximize nutrition and consciously move in order to realize sustained energy levels.

Naturally, we'll also discuss holistic beauty care. This is the healthy approach that we take to serve clients and answer their needs, relating directly to the synergy taking place between the health, fitness, and beauty fields.

As we continue our journey together, we will explore the path toward creating true beauty—the inner and outer beauty in first ourselves and then all others. Together we will discover ways to celebrate the sacredness of life, view every moment as a ritual for transformation, and ultimately see all that we experience as nurturing. Enjoy the journey!

> "There is a vitality, a life force, an energy, a quickening, that is translated through you into action, and because there is only one of you in all time, this expression is unique. And if you block it, it will never exist through any other medium and will be lost."
>
> *Martha Graham*

The Great Chain of Being

We as beauty professionals interact all the time with cherished clients, associates, managers, salon owners, vendors, and others. When you work from a higher level of consciousness, these interactions nurture great richness—for you as well as the receiver.

To achieve this higher level of consciousness, we strive to experience the multidimensional layers of our being. These layers within each person include body, mind, and spirit. In contemplative traditions, they make up the Great Chain of Being. In simple terms, this refers to three separate yet interrelated depths of insight. As you and I continue our journey, we will always try to view each situation through:

- the eye of the body, allowing us to see the material and sensual world around us.
- the eye of the mind, allowing us to see the conceptual, symbolic and linguistic world.
- the eye of contemplation, allowing us to see the spiritual and transcendental world.

Chapter One

Behold the Beauty Within

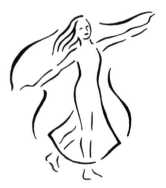

> " For behold, the kingdom
> of God is within you. "
> *Luke 17:21*

Do you know how beautiful you are? Yes, you! You *are* beautiful. Say this to yourself ten times. Right here, right now. I'll wait.

Okay. Now that you're back, think about how you felt as you affirmed your own beauty. Did you feel a spark of power? What if you used that spark to ignite a whole life filled with beauty? Imagine this tiny spark spiraling outward, casting a beautiful glow upon every thing and every person you see. Can you picture how glorious it would be to see all of life as interconnected and in this beautiful light of transformation? Once you achieve this realization, you will find more things to celebrate and fewer things to criticize. Now, if you will, imagine how those around you—family, friends, fellow beauty pros, as well as clients—will feel as they interact with you. How do you think these important people will react, dealing with you as a person who sees beauty in all the world and everyone in it? The residual effects of your self-realized beauty can be enormous.

In this chapter and throughout this book, we will explore ways to turn your spark into a radiant blaze. On a grand scale, this means achieving a sense of wholeness—a point where natural inner and outer beauty become inevitable. This wholeness represents a mystical moment when mind, body, and spirit—the three elements comprising your mindbody physiology—come together in harmonious balance. It is certain that this extreme beauty will positively radiate from you and cast its glow upon others.

> **" Toto, I've a feeling we're not in Kansas anymore. "**
>
> *Dorothy in* The Wizard of Oz

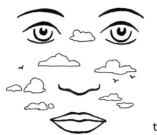

Wow! A lot of heavy talk. If it all seems a little out there right now, don't worry. Together we'll ignite that spark. For now, though, let's return to you. Let's talk some more about how beautiful you are!

As a beauty professional, you have a natural talent for appreciating all that is beautiful. Don't resist this ability. Affirm it. Spend the next few moments thinking about, appreciating, and writing down all that you find beautiful in yourself and your life. Let it flow unedited.

What would I write? Oh, something like . . .

I appreciate my legs, my curly hair, my nonjudgmental nature, my compassion for humanity and all of creation, my wonderful husband, my cherished family, my wonderful friends and dear clients, my dear pet companions, the air that I breathe, the nutritious food that I eat, my meditation and yoga practices, the first tomatoes out of the garden, my glorious scarlet red poppies opening for their brief spring fling, Friday-night martinis . . .

Now, you try it.

The Beauty I Appreciate.

_____

_____

_____

_____

_____

_____

_____

_____

"Come to the edge," he said.

They said, "We are afraid."

"Come to the edge," he said.

They came. He pushed them . . . and they flew.

Guillaume Apollinaire

Spread Your Wings and Fly

Now that you've affirmed how truly beautiful you are, let's spread out and see how far we can take this positive self-talk. Try approaching a finite period of time through positive affirmation, beginning with one 24-hour period.

Having trouble getting started? Try one of these affirmations:

- Each day is a new beginning—a fresh start.
- I'm alive and filled with vitality.
- Every day in every way, I'm getting better and better. (This is one of my favorite positive affirmations!)
- I'm a beauty professional because I enjoy making people feel better about themselves, and in turn I feel good about myself.

However you chose to express your affirmation, celebrate it with great clarity. Post it on your bathroom wall, embroider it on your clothing, dangle it from your car visor, write it in lipstick on your work-area mirror, tattoo it on your shoulder blade—do whatever it takes to revisit this intention. Before meditating in the morning, speak the words as a form of grace. Say it with relish! Smile as you say it. Sing it if you like. Ultimately you will program your subconscious to expect great things each day.

My affirmations.

_____

_____

_____

_____

> **Oh** God, help me to believe the truth about myself
> no matter how beautiful it is.
>
> *Macrina Wiederkehr from* A Grateful Heart

Places to put my affirmations so I may readily see them.

_____

_____

_____

_____

Positive Affirmation of Our Right Livelihood

At this point, you've positively affirmed your inner and outer beauty, as well as the fact that every day in every way, you're getting better and better. Now take this positive affirmation skill and try directing it to one specific issue—why you chose to enter the beauty profession. Positively reaffirm your original hopes, dreams, intentions, and goals. This is a great exercise for maintaining or rekindling the professional passion that originally beckoned you onto your chosen career path.

Here's how I might respond to the following question: Why the beauty profession?

- It offers loving relationships.
- It's my right livelihood—my destiny.
- I'm skilled at providing these services.
- I enjoy providing these services.
- It makes me feel alive and vibrant.
- It allows me artistic expression.
- It's filled with glamour.
- It's nurturing.
- It offers career growth.
- It works the left and right brain for ultimate creativity.

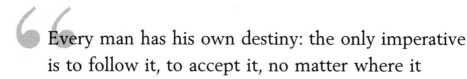

> Every man has his own destiny: the only imperative is to follow it, to accept it, no matter where it leads him.
>
> *Henry Miller*

Now you try.

Why the beauty profession?

_____

_____

_____

_____

_____

_____

_____

_____

_____

_____

_____

Go with the Flow

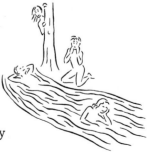

As you learn to behold a world filled with beauty, you will likely discover remarkable things in un-likely places. Maybe you'll find the uniqueness of your crooked nose suddenly quite appealing; perhaps you will find beauty in a new professional technique or management style; you may see beauty in a new attitude.

> *Only those who will risk going too far can possibly find out how far one can go.*
>
> T. S. Eliot

To help yourself positively affirm these beautiful hidden treasures, try imagining life as a river of energy and information that is forever changing, growing, and expanding. As the great philosopher Heraclitis said, "You can never step into the same river twice, because new water is always rushing in." It's important to remember that *new* refers to a fresh outlook on an old idea or a previously unknown concept.

Connecting with these amazing discoveries, however, may mean that you must release certain constraints or fears—concerns that prevent you from seeing or accepting something new. Fears can be strong, and letting go will probably be a gradual process. At first, you may only be able to peek through your doubt, as if dipping one toe into your river. Eventually, though, you can overcome any fear. One day you'll wake up with an overwhelming desire to plunge into your river and just go with the flow.

In order to let go of blocking fears, it might help to look more closely at *why* certain things scare you into numbness or tunnel vision. Many common fears stem from a general fear of change. Begin here. Ask yourself, "What is it about change that scares me?" Do any of the responses below hit home?

- *Fear of failure.* Accepting change means that you will need to deal with something new, and any time we handle the unfamiliar there is a possibility that we won't get it right the first time.
- *Fear of commitment.* With change comes the unknown, and committing to things unknown might lead to disappointment.
- *Fear of disapproval.* If we embrace change and consequently fail to produce the same old tried-and-true results, we might disappoint others and then need to deal with disapproval.
- *Fear of success.* Success is a wonderful thing, but admittedly it often brings with it added responsibilities, expectations, and goals.

Life-Force Energy

If we tap into our energy source, we can manifest all we desire and learn to work through change positively—fears be damned. We have the power to become the mystic, the sage, the shaman, playing without fear in this extremely fluid and changeable world. It all begins when we shift our consciousness toward our higher good and away from the many possible mis-

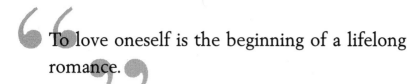

> To love oneself is the beginning of a lifelong romance.
>
> *Oscar Wilde*

steps along the way. We can choose to redirect the flow of our life-force energy toward our higher good (also known as our ultimate goals or our personal big picture), and away from the nearsighted lower base missteps we may experience. Returning to the fears we listed earlier, let's put a positive spin on them and shift our focus to a higher consciousness. Notice how I accomplish this through positive affirmations!

- I love experimentation, and I will use this creative drive to conquer my fear of failure.
- I love my ability to break larger goals into achievable interrelated steps, and I will use this tactic to conquer my fear of commitment.
- I love myself, and I will use this self-appreciation to conquer my fear of disapproval.
- I love to celebrate life, and I will use this joyous energy to conquer my fear of success.

Now you give it a try. List four reasons why you routinely fear or resist change. Then view these fears on a higher level of consciousness. How can each fear be redefined through a positive affirmation about yourself?

Four Reasons I Fear Change:

_____

_____

_____

_____

_____

_____

_____

> **Life shrinks or expands in proportion to one's courage.**
>
> *Anaïs Nin*

Four Positive Affirmations About Myself That Will Conquer My Fear of Change:

_____

_____

_____

_____

_____

Let Your Soul Write

Before you can decrease fear and increase confidence, you need to identify when, where, why, and how these emotions affect you. To help you do this, keep a journal each and every day. Write down whatever is on your mind—from the most mundane to the most bizarre thoughts and everything in between. This will prove tremendously cathartic for the soul, as it allows you to clear out the gunk, vent your feelings, and along the way make some important self-discoveries. For instance, you will probably spot repetition of thought. These are the areas in your life that need attention.

If struggling with a particular issue at your salon or spa, it's a good idea to keep your journal handy. In between clients or during a lunch break, write a few words about what's going on. Note your feelings and the sensations that these feelings create in your body and mind. If you have a difficult experience with a client or associate, talk it through—just you and your journal. And certainly, if you experience any form of fulfillment, exhilaration, love, and gratitude, note this as well. Acknowledging good feelings allows you to more readily see and feel the grace around you, and thus become an expression of this love and grace.

> If we all did the things we were capable of doing, we would literally astound ourselves.
>
> *Thomas Edison*

The Heart of the Matter

As we've seen, there are several ways to use your new ability to form positive affirmations. You can point this skill toward yourself alone, your life in general, or your chosen career path. We've even illustrated how positive affirmations can help reverse certain negative feelings, such as fear. On a much grander scale, positive affirmations represent one of your most remarkable tools for opening the heart and living life through a higher level of consciousness.

Western medicine typically sees the heart as a pump, beating on average 72 times per minute, roughly 100,000 times per 24-hour period. Our heart sends anywhere from 5 to 25 quarts of blood through 60,000 miles of blood vessels every minute and helps in circulating more than 100 million gallons in a lifetime.

Each heartbeat creates an electromagnetic wave that washes over every one of the 60 trillion cells in your body, and every single one of these cells—from the tips of our toes to the crown of our head—is being vibrated by your heart. The heartbeat's electromagnetic frequencies can be measured up to four feet away from the body. This may explain the expression *good vibrations,* as in good energy is flowing outward. The heartbeat's electromagnetic field might also explain why we sometimes sense *bad vibes* after only just entering a room. It may also explain why certain people have the power to cheer us up or calm us down. Good energy may flow outward from and surround these persons, and they may have mastered the ability to send these good vibrations out into the universe.

Mumbo jumbo or truth? Medical researchers are currently exploring the heart's ability to metabolize harmony, peace, and love. So far the answers point to truth! Some studies indicate that we humans possess incredible healing capabilities when we can learn to open our hearts. A study at the Institute of HeartMath, in Boulder Creek, California, asked one group of people to focus on feelings of love and appreciation whenever they began to feel angry or frustrated. After one month the participants' levels of DHEA, an anti-aging hormone, had increased 100 percent. Their levels of cortisol, a stress hormone, decreased 23 percent. It was also found that 80 percent of these people experienced slowed breathing rates and their hearts became synchronized with their breathing. In a control group there were no physical or hormonal changes. The researchers concluded, "There are a lot of implications for health. With feelings of love the inner systems synchronize. That affects your immune system, your hormones, and even cognitive performance."

Opening the Heart

Follow this simple practice to experience a shift in your outward flow of energy, moving away from your fears, toward your affirmation of all that is positive, and upward toward your higher consciousness.

Sit or lie down comfortably. With eyes closed, and breathing comfortably, place your palms against your chest. Bring all of your attention to your heart center. Now as you breathe, imagine that your breath is going directly into the center of your chest. Gently and tenderly hold the breath here for a count of four. As you breathe out, sense the breath moving into your palms, still placed on the chest. Each time you breathe in and out, feel the warmth and love being exchanged between the heart center

and your hands. You will begin to feel a sustained warmth and tenderness, expansion and delicacy. Begin to lift your hands away from the chest. Stay fully focused on the space between your hands and heart center. Intensify the feelings of warmth and love that you experience within this space. Continue to slowly make this space bigger, all the while focusing on the feelings of love and expansion.

Imagine broadcasting these feelings outward, toward anyone you choose. Sending out positive energy to others is a part of natural healing, and it is an ability that can propel the beauty professional to great success.

After trying the exercise above, you will find that there is a logical progression to this next one. Try hugging someone lightly (heart to heart)

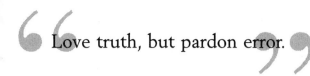

" Love truth, but pardon error. "

Voltaire

and tune in to the space between you both. Send this person your heart vibrations filled with love and warmth. Do this with a loved one, or if it's in your nature and style, with a client. This type of energy exchange can relax and revive you, and deepen your communion with others.

Other practices for opening the heart include breathing in your own or someone else's pain and breathing out love and peace. With each breath inhale the pain, then exhale love. You can also radiate light. Imagine a brilliant light in your heart center that is shining upon everyone and everything. If experiencing a conflict or difficulty with someone, consider this bright light as a sort of spotlight. Keep broadening the area upon which your spotlight shines, until finally it illuminates the conflict. Look closely to see what this conflict teaches you. Be thankful for this learning experience.

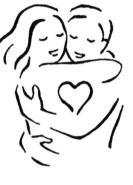

Good Medicine

Remember this one truth—you are a healer, a shaman. Your capacity for healing knows no bounds. Our creativity, our actions, our attitude, our manner of speech, our behavior, our touch, our words, and, yes, our love—they all have potential to heal. This wonderful power begins with the care you give yourself. Take those fears you have about change and turn them around until you become focused on all the good and healthy elements inherent in change. Once you harness the ability to heal your own fears, then you can begin working from the heart, sending love and kindness out to others. Everything that we do within the beauty profession is about loving communion with others. We have the power to bring good medicine to everyone we touch—beginning with ourselves. It is our dharma—our purpose in life.

> **I shut my eyes in order to see.**
>
> *Paul Gauguin*

Dharma Is More Than a Sitcom Character

What is dharma, you ask? Dharma is our purpose in life. We all have our own unique talents, and when shared with others these gifts can bring us to an experience of blissful spirit. We are constantly discovering new ways in which to express our dharma, sometimes from a personal perspective, sometimes from a professional standpoint, and oftentimes from a perspective that brilliantly blends all our personas.

Write down your unique talents. Perhaps you have a knack for making others feel comfortable. Maybe you have a gentle touch that puts people at ease. How about your ability to make others laugh? Certainly you want to include your imagination and creativity! Now go a step farther and visualize how your unique gifts help others. Note the similarities between your dharma list and the list of things you love about yourself (page 12). Do you see overlapping entries? Interesting!

_____

_____

_____

_____

_____

_____

_____

_____

_____

_____

_____

_____

> When I am working on a problem, I never think about beauty. I only think about how to solve the problem. But when I have finished, if the solution is not beautiful, I know it is wrong.
>
> *Buckminster Fuller (1895–1983)*

From the Past Comes Present-Moment Awareness

To keep your heart open—flowing parallel to life's river of energy and information—you need to cleverly maintain a sharp focus on the present. Ironically, one of your best tools for living in the present is remembering the past.

For example, in order to positively affirm the beauty in your chosen career, you might need to review the original reasons you entered this field.

Take a few moments now to remember the literal steps as well as emotional inspiration that brought you to your calling as a beauty professional.

What challenges did you face while training for your work?

_____

_____

_____

_____

What challenges did you overcome?

_____

_____

_____

_____

Why did you bother to overcome these challenges, fears, and obstacles?

_____

_____

_____

_____

Remember, rekindle, and reaffirm all the choices you made long ago or perhaps just recently. Embrace your destiny as a beauty and wellness professional and as a healer. Be thankful for having come this far and for all the lessons learned along the way.

_____

_____

_____

_____

Creative Visualization into the Future

While recalling previous passions can help strengthen present awareness, forecasting yourself into the future may also prove a valuable tool. I refer to visualization, the next logical step after mastering positive affirmation. Visualization positively affirms your hopes, dreams, and goals. When done from the heart, it can help you manifest the perfect job, harmonious work relationships, exquisite well-being, and, when collectively done, even world peace.

Distinct evidence exists that healing through visualization has been around for more than 40,000 years! Early cave paintings in France show pictures of powerful animals—such as buffalo—drawn next to stick figures of injured people. Ancient man drew pictures pleading with the gods for rain, good harvests, relief from disease, and life after death. Symbolism such as this is still used today in Native American shamanism. Today sports physiologists teach Olympic athletes to envision every nuance of tomorrow's performance. Physicians teach patients to envision health.

Creative visualization, sometimes called guided imagery, is a practice that you can use anytime, anywhere to form desirable images in your mind. This might mean visualizing a beautiful scene in a relaxing place. Allow your mind to see every detail of this special place. Engage all your senses and become intimate with every nuance—the life forms, colors, aromas, sound, and textures. Stay with this visualization for as long as you want. You will feel incredibly relaxed afterwards.

Believers find that visualization can effectively transform behavior or thought patterns, cutting through the chatter in our heads and leading us to a higher level of consciousness, where mind, body, and spirit become one. For example, that beautiful scene I just described could be your destination when faced with a perplexing challenge. Taking this imagery a step farther: visualize yourself in this relaxing place, sitting against a tree trunk and imagining a solution to your problem. Let yourself see the desired outcome to any challenge.

There are so many instances where creative visualization might work. You might visualize letting go of a destructive relationship, presenting a new idea, meeting someone for the first time with grace and calm, performing a service on a client, managing stress, or overcoming fear. Practice this technique often. Visualization is a powerful technique for programming your subconscious. You may manifest what you visualize!

In your mind's eye see yourself doing exactly what it is you feel like doing. Eating an ice-cream cone? Walking along the beach? Playing with a child? Whatever makes you happy is precisely what you should be seeing. Little by little, zoom your image outward, until you have all five senses engaged in this imagery. When you feel comfortable with this part of the exercise, you're ready for the tough stuff. Next you want to envision yourself fulfilling deep desires or goals. Place your intention as well as your attention where you want your consciousness to move. Think as big as you want! Let your creative visualization program your subconscious to follow a desired path. Be careful what you wish for! Creative visualization is a powerful tool toward taking action, and wishes can come true!

> " All substance is energy in motion. It lives and flows. Money is symbolically a golden, flowing stream of concretized vital energy. "
>
> *From* The Magical Work of the Soul

There's No Time Like the Present

While recalling the past often helps rekindle present-moment awareness, and forecasting yourself into the future often helps turn dreams into reality, too much of either is not a good thing. Do you sometimes feel like your passion's left the building? Maybe it's because you're so frantically working toward the future or living in the past you've forgotten how to appreciate the present. Try bringing your focus back to the here and now. For some, this may mean taking a day off and enjoying time without a purpose or goal. For others, returning to the present might involve simplifying the to-do list. Learn to say no! This may require quelling a possible fear of disappointing others, but the result will be more time to actually see and enjoy what you're doing as you do it! Do whatever it takes to feel passionate about today. When our passion burns brightly, we have the energy to change, create, heal, and manifest.

Prosperity Consciousness

Everything we've explored so far will hopefully help you in loving yourself, your career, and your universe. When you can positively affirm a deep passion for all three dimensions, and indeed blend the three areas seamlessly into the fabric of your life, you've achieved the most wonderful kind of success there is.

My dear friend and mentor Leo Passage taught me, "Do what you love and success will follow." The question is "What do we mean by success?" For me, the definition of success—or prosperity—is twofold. You can measure success by the degree of satisfaction you feel deep in your soul, and you can also characterize success by the number of dollars in your bank account.

Each form of achievement is real, admirable, and viable. When you achieve balance between both definitions, you achieve prosperity consciousness.

So, returning to Leo's wise advice for a moment, you can do what you love to achieve financial success, and you can do what you love to feed your soul. They indeed can be one and the same! Your work can feed your soul, and it can bring you great financial success. It depends on your consciousness, and having your heart in the right place.

You have to decide for yourself what will brighten your soul. I can make suggestions, though. In a hurting world, couldn't every one of us share our prosperity with those less fortunate? Go to a local homeless shelter and cut hair or give massages. Contact a women's shelter and help these people face the job market looking their absolute best. Volunteer at a local hospice. If you give back as much as you get, you will find yourself creating a most rewarding cycle, experiencing the joy of giving while at the same time attracting the money that you need to live simply and comfortably.

1. Identify some of the things you could accomplish with financial success (pay off bills, buy a condo, purchase a new car, start a business).

_____

_____

_____

_____

_____

2. Identify some of the ways financial success makes you feel (exhilarated, secure, free, proud, joyous, self-fulfilled, triumphant).

_____

_____

_____

_____

_____

> 66 God is a comedian playing to an audience too afraid to laugh. 99
>
> *Voltaire*

3. Identify some of the ways you could achieve spiritual success (showing loving-kindness to all, donating your talents to the less fortunate, volunteering at a shelter, organizing a dress-for-success day at a local women's shelter).

_____

_____

_____

_____

_____

4. Identify some of the ways spiritual success makes you feel (exhilarated, secure, free, proud, joyous, self-fulfilled, triumphant).

_____

_____

_____

_____

_____

Can you see the repetition of feelings in lists number 2 and number 4? I think you get my point!

The Child Within

Positive affirmations, overcoming fears, creative visualization, respectful and responsible prosperity consciousness . . . these are all very grown-up concepts. Before you let yourself become too adult, however, I implore you—protect and hold dear your child within.

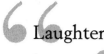
Laughter is the shortest distance between two people.

Victor Borge

Generally speaking, children have not yet had time to let an inner censor take over, that mighty reflex that frowns on new ideas, prohibits unbridled laughter, forbids the heartfelt tear, and scoffs at business-*not-as-usual*.

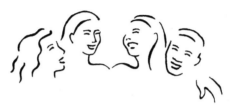

There are actually laughing clubs springing up around the world. The Healing Works Laugh Club, with around 80 chapters nationwide, offers its members laughing exercises that flow into spontaneous laughter. Consider adding a laugh class to your salon or spa menu. Or start a salon-based laughter club. Not only will you be providing a little levity, but you may also cure what ails a client!

Laughter has definite healing properties, creating physiological changes as the action triggers a release of natural feel-good chemicals into the body. It helps fend off disease by activating immunological cells; it elevates brain awareness and increases levels of natural pain-killing opioids; and it is proven to reduce stress hormones. Laughter may not always be the best medicine, but it sure comes close.

One Final Thought

I hope that you now see how one tiny positive feeling about one tiny element can spiral out to give you a more beautiful, rewarding view of the entire world. In turn, I hope you understand how this magical view of the universe brings greater health and beauty to all who cross your path.

Embracing this insight, let's return to that question I posed in the book's introduction: How may I serve? For perhaps the first time in your life, I invite you to ask *yourself* this question. Respect your answer. Now consider how your answer will reach out to serve personal and professional people in your world. Remember, today more than ever, our personal and professional lives have become one.

> The Master in the art of living
> makes little distinction between
> his work and his play,
> his labor and his leisure,
> his mind and his body,
> his education and his recreation,
> his love and his religion.
> He hardly knows which is which.
> He simply pursues his vision of
> excellence
> in whatever he does,
> leaving others to decide
> whether he is working or playing.
> To him his is always doing both.
>
> Zen Buddhist text

Become a master in the art of living. Write down areas in your life that become happily confused—areas where you are literally working, but it sure feels like play!

Don't hold back, censor or edit. Use your new knowledge of self, but also let your inner child run free. Be seduced by the exhilaration of it all. This is what life is meant to feel like. Oh, rapturous joy.

_____

_____

_____

_____

_____

_____

_____

_____

_____

_____

_____

_____

_____

_____

Notes:

Chapter Two

Taking Care of the Caregiver

Be really whole, and all things will come to you.

Lao Tzu

There are plenty of books out there to help you better care for the beauty salon or spa client, improve your people skills, balance a salon budget, or manage a spa staff, but while you are busy learning how to be an effective caregiver, who is taking care of the caregiver? Who is taking care of you?

When you find and nurture the spirit within yourself, you've actually taken the first step toward providing better care to others. Remember the start of this book, when we discussed that spark? When you encourage your own emotional growth, and maintain exquisite health and wellness, the results can only be fulfillment, happiness, and true beauty. In addition to nurturing your own well-being, these sorts of wonderful emotions can not be contained. Like rays of sunshine, they burst from your soul and shine upon all others. It is undeniable the influence we have when we choose to care for ourselves first.

To better understand what I mean, review the following series of choices, first considering how each option affects you and then how each option affects others. Every day we have the freedom to choose how we express our thoughts, attitudes, and actions. We may greet the world with serenity, humility, and rapturous joy, or we may choose to approach the day with agitation, disrespect, short-temperedness, and impatience. How do you feel when you approach a situation with joy? How does a client or associate feel when you approach a situation with joy? The decision to approach every circumstance today with a positive outlook may stem

> We're all equally divine, but we're all at different stages of actualizing our divine potential. The fullest expression of our divine potential is to be someone who helps others actualize their potential.
>
> *Gordon Davidson, president of the*
> *Center for Visionary Leadership*

from self-care—it makes *me* feel better about *myself*—but in the end, this attitude serves self, neighbor, fellow beauty pros, and client.

As you continue being kind to yourself—taking care of the caregiver— so too will goodness continue radiating from you, flowing outward as pure vibrating energy. We exchange vital energy with each client we touch, affecting every relationship in profound ways. If we send out good energy and it is accepted, we can step into and influence the aura of each client. You will no longer be bound by salon or spa services, but instead you will be empowered to gently guide your clients toward defining their personal sense of style and, in essence, enhance their self-esteem. You can create the ultimate beauty and wellness experience for clients, and after they leave your salon or spa, they take with them the magic of an encounter with you. How cool is that?

Soulful Work

So let's get down to the business of making your business better. Let's figure out how to take care of you! In life we all have basic needs and drives to find fulfillment and happiness. These needs progress from what would be considered lower-level needs upward along the ladder of success toward the higher-level needs. When our lower-level needs are met, we are more able to open up and have our fullest human potential shine through. As stated in Abraham Maslow's Hierarchy of Needs, an upward progression in these needs might look like this:

- *Physical needs*—nutritious food, rejuvenating sleep, a roof over our heads, adequate clothing.
- *Financial security*—a reliable job that can support our physical needs as well as future plans.
- *Social needs*—relationships that provide love, companionship, and a sense of belonging.

> It is not how much we do, but how much love we put into the doing. And it is not how much we give but how much love we put into the giving. To God there is nothing small.
>
> *Mother Theresa*

- *Self-esteem*—recognition, appreciation, and status, all necessary to foster self-confidence and self-worth.

Working through these needs clears a path for deeper concentration on the highest level of needs—self-actualization and creative fulfillment. Now we can begin working from the heart, moving forward to achieve our fullest human potential.

Again, I can not stress enough, your personal success as a human being helps you succeed brilliantly in serving your clients. Your poise, emotional intelligence, eye contact, listening skills, manner of speech, touch, and sensitivity all depend so fiercely on the level of grace with which you approach your own life, make choices, and enhance your own well-being. As you achieve your own creative potential, so too will the person sitting in your chair move toward realizing his or her creative self. This is beauty and wellness integration at its best.

Finding Your Best Answers

There is a profound spiritual renaissance taking place in our culture. We see it in the many ways our society searches for true meaning—in relationships, careers, existence. Are you part of this renaissance? Are there days you ask yourself, "What am I doing this for? I *know* I can I feel more fulfilled than this"? The most reassuring part about all these queries is that the answers do exist, deep within you. Pay attention to your heart and soul. This is where your natural inner voice comes from, and if you listen carefully, it will supply the answers to your questions. When you hear your own inner voice, you will experience a spiritual awakening. Trivial matters will be replaced with a sense of awe. You will feel and send out irrepressible joy, vitality, creativity, peace, and yes, love.

When we tap into the wellspring of these feelings, everything we do and everyone we meet—casually, professionally, or on an intimate level—will, to some degree, mirror our positive energy.

> I think most of us are looking for a calling, not a job. Most of us, like the assembly line worker, have jobs that are too small for our spirit. Jobs are not big enough for people.
>
> *Nora Watson, interviewed by*
> *Studs Terkel in* Working

You should know that achieving your higher-level needs—creative fulfillment and self-actualization—is more possible today than ever before. It all hinges on the paradigm shift occurring within the professional beauty industry as well as within the beauty professional. As this book continues, we'll study in greater depth this shift and its enormous benefits, but for now let me simply define it as a move away from our old title of *beautician* and toward new titles such as *designer, artist, creator, dreamweaver.* In fact, the standards by which we define our career scope have broadened so dramatically that we now find beauty professionals using their talents in the health and fitness fields as well as in the beauty arena. So you can understand why it is of paramount importance to find your center and stay grounded in the value of your work. For the first time, you have career choices to make that can and will allow you to say, "I *know* I can feel as if I'm fulfilling my every need and destiny . . . and I also know precisely how to sustain this feeling."

A Beautiful Progression

The new spiritual vision within the beauty profession is dynamically and energetically moving forward. Whether you realize it yet or not, you have chosen a career that can become your life's work, a career rather than job, a calling.

This remarkable vision begins with the natural integration of health, fitness, and beauty. Since this process began in the '70s, I and many others have tried to stay at its forefront. My hope is that every beauty professional will become an active participant in this evolution, considering the wealth of opportunity this unfolding affords.

The beauty professional may be a hair designer, makeup artist, esthetician, massage therapist, herbalist, retail specialist, yoga or meditation instructor, salon coordinator, or business manager or have one of many additional career titles. The beauty professional can work solo, in a health

> Let us not go over old ground, let us rather prepare for what's to come.

Cicero

practitioner's office, side by side with a physician, in a wellness spa, or in a hair salon.

When I went to beauty school back in the mid-1970s, it was not unusual to meet classmates who were attending beauty school until something better came along—like a husband to support them! I also met fellow students who only wanted to cut hair so they could earn money for traditional college tuition. These reasons for becoming a licensed beauty professional aren't wrong, they're simply short-lived.

During my school days, I did meet students like myself—people focused on long-term career goals. We chose to become beauty professionals because this career option enlivened, inspired, stimulated, fulfilled, and touched us like nothing else. Largely because of the huge career potential within the beauty profession, today there are more and more seriously dedicated beauty professionals graduating from cosmetology school as well as many other beauty- and wellness-aligned vocational schools. I urge you to welcome with open hearts and minds every one of these fellow professionals. They are not competitors but rather allies. We should unite with great commitment and zealousness in our goal to push even farther the boundaries that once limited our profession.

This book is a sacred celebration of our occupational choice, a choice that has moved far, far away from yesteryear's title of cut-and-curl beautician and into a professional arena filled with infinite possibilities. It's all about paddling down our river of information and knowledge with an open mind, great expectations, and the right attitude.

Do You Guru?

To fully embrace the wonders of our chosen career, you need the right attitudes. The first feeling you should examine pertains to mentoring. A mentor is a teacher, a guide, a guru—someone who knows or does all the things you want to know or do. It is important for all of us to seek out potential mentors in our life. With tremendous gratefulness, we should hang on their every word and watch what they do.

Some of us shy away from seeking guidance because we think we can do it better ourselves. Balderdash. We all need help. It's all about learning,

> We must become the change we want to see.
>
> *Mahatma Gandhi*

the one thing that will never become obsolete. The healthiest one among us is the person who realizes that getting help is not a sign of weakness or ineptitude, but rather a sign of real desire, dedication to this desire, and a drive to achieve this desire sooner than later. If you must, consider asking for help as a shortcut. Who wouldn't like to achieve financial and spiritual success while they're still fully able to enjoy it!

Others might think it's embarrassing to seek out a mentor. Get rid of this attitude right now. Asking for help is an enormous compliment. Think how you would feel if someone said, "When you give a body wave, it always looks so incredibly healthy and natural. How do you do that?" You'd feel pretty darn great, that's how you'd feel. Now go find someone you admire and give them the greatest compliment of all—ask for their guidance.

I want to remind you that a mentor can help with personal skills as well as technical skills. Being a beauty professional has always been about developing relationships with clients, and if you feel this is an area that someone else elegantly commands, ask this person to share their wisdom.

Who Do You Admire?

Take a few reflective moments to think about individuals who touch you on a deep level and single out someone you would like to learn more from. This can be an individual you work with or someone you came to know through a seminar, a television show, or a book.

Make a resolution to connect with your mentor. March up to this person, express your admiration, and ask for help. If this option is not doable, write a letter. It's a little less predictable than face-to-face conversation, but there's always a chance that you might get a response.

You could also seek a position at one of the many salons with mentorship programs already in place. Senior stylists guide the newbies, and it's a terrific opportunity to begin your career and continue your education all at once.

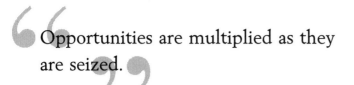

Opportunities are multiplied as they are seized.

Sun Tzu

Don't forget to think outside the perm rod box. Depending on which direction you see your career moving, you might find a mentor in the medical community, the music community, the fitness community, or the fashion community!

People I admire (name, business address, business phone number):

_____

_____

_____

_____

_____

_____

_____

_____

_____

_____

_____

_____

_____

Just as I urge you to seek a mentor, I also urge you to become one. Maybe you see someone struggling with a concept. Maybe they're one of those persons who feels uncomfortable asking for help. Offer your insight and knowledge. Given kindly and from the heart, your suggestions will most likely be accepted with gratitude.

> *Each of us makes his own weather. We determine the color of the skies in the emotional universe that we inhabit.*
>
> Fulton J. Sheen

Take Out the Trash

We humans tend to walk through life carrying a lot of useless baggage—including past hurts, resentments, and sadnesses. It is so important to let these unhealthy emotions go, before all this garbage creates fragmentation within us and leaves us confused and depleted. In Chapter One we

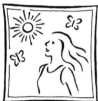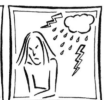

talked about the importance of present moment awareness, once you hone this skill, you will be more likely to leave the past and exuberantly enjoy the present. This is vital in order to clear a path for spiritual evolution, not to mention beauty and wellness.

The Emotional Clearing Process

Hopefully you've now decided to take out the trash, letting past unhappiness go in order to fully enjoy the present. Now you are ready to take full responsibility for your own feelings. Tackle any unhealthy attitudes that may be locked up inside you. It's going to be difficult to let some of this garbage go—anxiety, guilt, depression, anger, malaise, sadness—after all, any one of these attitudes and emotions may have been a part of you for so very long. Maybe this exercise will help.

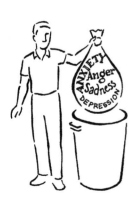

- Identify one negative emotion in a very matter-of-fact way.
- Pinpoint the causes of the emotion.
- State the reasons for this emotion or write them down, as clearly as possible.
- Pay attention to the emotion. Witness it fully.
- What are the physical sensations that this emotion creates in your body? Does the emotion create a backache, stomach ache, or headache?)
- Now work toward releasing the emotion and any painful body sensations.

Once you release the emotion, celebrate! Take a luxurious bath. Go for a luscious walk through the local park or forest preserve. Prepare and eat a nourishing meal. Listen to your favorite music. Get a massage.

When you have finished this entire process, tune in to your body and mind. Do you notice a shift in attitude? Congratulations! You just gave yourself a tremendous gift. Use this process to dispel other unhealthy emotions. Give yourself a whole pile of gifts!

Resolving Conflict

Some emotions are nearly impossible to get rid of, largely because of their spontaneous and unpredictable nature. (Anger is one of these emotions. Love is another, but of course this is a good thing!)

In addition, you will sometimes find yourself in situations where you must manage not only your own spontaneous emotions but also unpredictable emotions from other persons involved in a particular scenario. To more healthfully deal with emotional clinches you may have with others, try the following guidelines, offered originally at a wonderful website, www.angermgmt.com:

Phase One

1. Identify the negative behavior.
2. Resist the temptation to take the angry remarks seriously, as if they were valid observations instead of irrational statements.
3. Don't try to reason with the person while they're acting unreasonably.
4. Try to identify and understand the underlying reasons for their anger. This will help you empathize instead of arguing with them.

Phase Two

1. Validate their anger with statements such as "I don't blame you for being angry." Showing that you respect them as a person instead of pointing out imperfections may quickly cool them down.
2. Give them a choice of talking to you or writing a memo after they have calmed down. Ask them to include any ways you might help remedy the situation.
3. Stand your ground, but don't become hostile. Agree with them that it would be nice if they could get what they want, but don't give in if you're not comfortable with their solution.

> Compassion is the ultimate and most meaningful embodiment of emotional maturity. It is through compassion that a person achieves the highest peak and the deepest reach in his or her search for self-fulfillment.
>
> *Arthur Jersild*

Have Compassion

In a time when road rage, air rage, desk rage, and downright incivility surround us, what can we do to bring peace and harmony into our lives? You can begin by having compassion for others. I guarantee this kindness will come around to reward you richly. Begin today by opening your heart and feeling tenderness for others—whether it's someone you work with, a homeless person on the street, or a spider crawling along the wall. Go to that place of your pure potentiality, that place of your higher consciousness, and commune with your spirit.

As I've continued my study of compassion, one of my most amazing discoveries involves the fact that no one is right or wrong—they're just different. So instead of saying, "You are wrong!" try asking yourself "Where is this person coming from?" This thought process can dramatically change your interactions. When you understand where someone is coming from, you automatically become less judgmental. When you become less judgmental, you become more tolerant. When you become more tolerant, you are more readily able to forgive. And when you are more forgiving, you are more readily able to love unconditionally.

Every single person we connect with has a story to tell. Everyone has lived through a unique succession of experiences. We have all received different amounts of nurturing, support, and guidance. A person's upbringing contributes to creating his or her level of consciousness. It explains the circumstances that brought a person to a certain place. Perhaps it is not so much that you are right and they are wrong, as that the two of you are coming from different levels of consciousness and understanding. For unknown reasons, some people awaken sooner than others. One thing is certain, we'll all get there.

> **Be kind. Everyone you meet is carrying a heavy burden.**
>
> *Unknown*

Forgiveness Is Good for the Mind, Body, and Soul

To err is human, to forgive is smarter . . . at least this is what studies suggest. Growing evidence shows that those inclined to forgive enjoy better physical and mental health than those prone to grudges. In one study, adults were asked to use either unforgiving or forgiving imagery as they thought about someone who had wronged them. Those thinking "no mercy" experienced a significant rise in heart rate and blood pressure, while their moods worsened. Those who imagined showing forgiveness had healthier vital statistics, and who knows how much peace of mind.

Too Much Caring Can Be Wearing

My mother has told me on more than one occasion, "Mary Beth, you can't save the entire world." Maybe Mom's right. Maybe my deep compassion for people, animals, and all of creation is on occasion detrimental to my own well-being. Compassion has tremendous value in our lives, but know that it can also be carried to the extreme. Experts call this compassion fatigue—likened to post-traumatic stress syndrome. We as beauty and wellness consultants need to protect ourselves—show some compassion for our own energy—if we hope to have compassion for our clients.

If you sense that you are on the verge of compassion fatigue, it may be necessary to pull back, take a vacation, visit a spa. If you are experiencing full-blown compassion fatigue, talk to your primary care physician, a therapist, or anyone else who can help bring you through this episode successfully, with your caring, compassionate, and energetic self restored.

You're a Teacher

In this chapter we've discussed several ways to satisfy your highest-level needs, more specifically your life long need for self-actualization and creative fulfillment. My final suggestion may surprise you. Learn to think of yourself as a teacher and not a salesperson. You should be constantly *teaching* clients about what it is you have to offer. Share your expertise and sacred knowledge. In this way you are providing better client service, of course, but you are also cultivating your soul through your heart's true work. You are valuing your own knowledge and experience by deeming it worthy, interesting, and valuable enough to share. On a simplistic level, it all comes down to this: by giving you will receive.

Become fully proficient and knowledgeable in your chosen craft, integrating this knowledge into your heart and mind. Share what you know as a beauty professional and educator with great enthusiasm and vitality. In doing so, you will be sharing your passion for beauty, truth, and goodness, and everyone you touch physically, mentally, and spiritually will take away an experience of love and beauty. While our motivation should be to serve others, such good and pure intentions also bring additional rewards—fame, money, even adoration. While I won't lie to you and say that these various forms of recognition would not be nice, I'd like to stress that the self-fulfillment and self-actualization that also result are even better!

Cultivating the Soul at Work

When we allow ourselves to experience bliss and happiness, we radiate and thus share this deep satisfaction with all others. I would like to share the following spiritual checklist. Read it carefully, adapt it to your own higher-level needs, and then go captivate the world!

- Learn to think of your work as a calling, a profession, a career. This will help you feel professionally fulfilled.
- Keep a clear focus on your life's meaning and mission. Get in touch with your heart and what you care about most deeply.
- Know that the essence of a beauty professional is caring and that you make a difference in other lives.

"We are on a quest, individually and collectively, to create wholeness within ourselves and within all of our life, to find it within ourselves and to release it— a process of communion and education. What is created will not be separation, conflict and diversity among peoples, but wholeness, oneness, peace, a new earth for humankind that reflects the oneness and wholeness of the earth that has always been."

David Spangler

- Keep your professional passion alive. Revisit and reflect often on why you wanted to become a beauty professional.
- Master what you do on the highest level possible and on a continuing basis. This allows you to feel the deepest sense of accomplishment.
- Value your talents, skills, and abilities.
- Confront your fears and all other negative feelings, release them, and move on . . . take a few risks.
- Tune in to yourself. Meditate to quiet the overactive mind. Breathe deeply. Go for a walk. Eat nourishing, whole foods. Hear what your inner voice says and then heed this message in order to find your center.
- Cultivate present-moment awareness, and appreciate the positive, nourishing aspects of any situation—good or bad.
- Be compassionate with yourself and others. When we forgive rather than judge, we learn to love.
- Choose to be peaceful inside, even in the face of crisis. Step back, relax, and connect with life's bigger picture.
- Be a teacher and share your knowledge. You will nurture others and in the process progress toward self-actualization.
- Focus on the wholeness of life rather than fragments, and don't lose sight of what is truly important.
- Practice creative visualization and positive affirmations. Both actions help define and ultimately manifest your desires.
- Engage fully with all persons you meet. Listen to their stories, look deep into their eyes, and see the soul that resides there.

Notes:

Taking Care of the Caregiver

Chapter Three

Beauty in Mind, Body, and Spirit

> Beauty is truth, truth beauty; that is all ye know on earth, and all ye need to know.
>
> *John Keats*

As a beauty professional, I urge you to consider the age-old cliché "Beauty is only skin deep." I ask you to delve way below the surface until you hit the deeper meaning: physical shapes made of skin, cartilage, bone, and muscle as they are arranged on the human body represent only one layer of beauty, and a human's total beauty continues to evolve below the surface of the skin, encompassing one's attitudes, outlook, and connection to spirit.

Phew. That's a long sentence, and definitely not the kind of stuff that makes for a nice, neat proverb! But you get my drift. You also now have the point of this chapter: beauty is a very personal and spiritual entity.

To begin your blissful journey toward a spiritual connection with beauty, I suggest you examine your own interpretation of that which is beautiful. We all have a private and personal definition of beauty, and we all want to be this beauty, surround ourselves with this beauty, and create this beauty.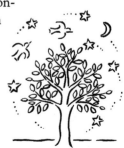

What do you find beautiful? Begin by considering anything that brings you joy. These are things you wouldn't mind experiencing any moment of any day.

You might also want to consider challenges, for even a formidable task or situation can potentially teach us something beautiful.

As you become spiritually tuned in to your own definition of beauty, you will begin to see and experience more beauty. It's a wonderfully self-perpetuating cycle. So, tune in! This may mean going to an art museum, tooling around the garden, driving along country roads, making love with your significant other, running along the ocean, eating a sumptuous meal, or contemplating the stars.

To fully appreciate beauty, we need to first experience beauty. Remember, this begins with our openhearted perception. This is how we learn to personally and most profoundly define beauty. So go out into the world and consciously seek out beauty, relish it, learn from it. List here experiences, places, and people that have brought and may continue to bring beauty into your life. These are things you should look for, again and again and again! If there are things you *think* you'd find beautiful, add them to your list as well. Before you know it, you will begin to see the beauty in every single nuance of your world.

Beautiful experiences I've had:

_____

_____

_____

_____

_____

_____

_____

_____

_____

_____

_____

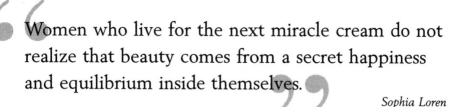

> "Women who live for the next miracle cream do not realize that beauty comes from a secret happiness and equilibrium inside themselves."
>
> *Sophia Loren*

Experiences I think I'll find beautiful—experiences I will try to have soon:

_____

_____

_____

_____

_____

_____

_____

_____

_____

_____

_____

Approach Beauty with Attitude

For the beauty professional, it is doubly important to understand the full depth of beauty. We are in the profession of seeing, finding, and creating beauty. Every action we take as beauty professionals is devoted to a beautification experience—whether cutting hair, performing a facial, giving a massage, sweeping hair, serving tea, folding towels, or soothing a client's tension.

The effectiveness of any one action depends on our approach and our attitude. We choose the energy that we cause to flow into this experience of beauty. If we are self-centered, ego driven, and distracted, and mindlessly approach our actions, these movements will help no one. Be humble, and learn to give of yourself to another. Open your heart. Teach yourself to commune with clients. Look into their eyes and see the soul that resides there. You have the power to change a person's day, life, attitude, and self-esteem. You should know, too, that these transformations can only be realized when you are fully present with yourself.

Extreme Self-Care

The integration of beauty and wellness means choosing a path of extreme self-care. This does not mean being extremely careful about eating a power bar for lunch instead of a hamburger and fries! And it does not mean adding a neck massage to your shampoo treatment or stocking organic personal care products in your salon or spa. While these steps all play a small part in the definition of beauty and wellness integration, none of these efforts alone can turn your business into a spa! It goes so much farther and deeper.

Beauty and wellness integration is about a holistic way of thinking—your attitude! It is about making choices that allow glorious life force energy to flow freely through us and around us. This holistic way of living allows our truest beauty to shine through, and when we feel beautiful—inside and out—we naturally enhance our self-esteem, optimism, and resiliency.

One attitude that beautifully supports holistic thinking is optimism—our ability to see the best in everyone and everything. It gives us the perceptiveness to see a beautiful and good world, and to learn and grow from all we experience—positive or negative.

Let me give you a single example. Perhaps you've had something stolen from you. Naturally, this feels like a violation. If you can shift your perception to that of detachment, you may be able to see that whoever took this thing must have needed it more than you! Eliciting this type of energy within can prevent feelings of grief, sadness, or victimization. I don't mean to belittle that object stolen from you, or deny that you deserve to feel a moment of anger. But by quickly getting over it and instead focusing on a feeling of optimism, you will get through the situation much more quickly, and you will come out of it with your mind-body health in a much better place.

Beyond enjoying emotional benefits, optimists have higher levels of natural killer cell activity, so they tend to be more capable of fighting disease. It is scientifically proven that positive affirmations raise the immune system's white cell blood count. Amazing! Optimists also have lower levels of the stress hormone cortisol. In addition, a long-term study conducted by the Mayo Clinic suggests that optimists outlive their pessimistic counterparts. Approximately 850 people were given a personality survey in the '60s that helped classify them as optimists, pessimists, or both. Looking at the subjects thirty years later, researchers found that pessimists had a 19 percent higher risk of death. Now pessimists have something else to worry about!

Optimism is also key to developing tremendous resiliency—the ability to take what life hands you and get through it, get over it, and get on. It's the ability to be challenged but not break down. Some New Age thinkers are calling resiliency the *it* skill of the new millennium.

What makes a person resilient? Most importantly, it is an ability to feel connected to others. Resilient people tend to be self-reliant, flexible, and capable of nurturing personal relationships. These people are also able to learn from bad events, as opposed to feeling like a victim.

We all experience misfortunes and losses—it is part of our destiny—and setbacks can serve to strengthen our will. Be the optimist. Allow yourself to bounce back. You can't stop enjoying the wonder and miracle of life. Choosing to be the resilient optimist comes from a deep sense of connection with spirit. In connecting with spirit through meditation, creative visualization, and positive affirmations, you will wind your way along this path called life. And remember to take side trips as needed along this path, seeking out support from friends, family, or qualified professionals. I personally have some confidants who help me see a brighter and lighter side to some of the shadows lurking in my life. This connection and communion with others can possibly help stave off life-depleting pessimism or depression.

Turn stressful situations that routinely confront you into something absurd. Enlarge the absurdity in your mind until you can no longer resist a good guffaw. My example: This rush-hour traffic is horrible. I'm going to be stuck in traffic for the rest of my life and starve to death, and they'll find me here half-eaten by wild animals. Of course, my scenario is ridiculous. It's impossible. The worst thing that will happen is that I'll be 15 minutes late for my meeting. But making up this absurd story helps me reevaluate my level of frustration. Is it really justified? I mean, it's not like I'm going to be eaten by wild animals.

> Health and disease don't just happen to us. They are active processes issuing from inner harmony or disharmony, profoundly affected by our states of consciousness, our ability or inability to flow with experience.
>
> *Marilyn Ferguson*

That would be something to panic over. Now you try. Think of the last situation that caused you to feel a huge amount of pessimistic or negative emotion. Make up a silly ending to your story and have a good laugh. I bet the next time a similar situation rears its ugly head, you'll recall your absurd story and feel much better about the whole thing!

_____

_____

_____

_____

_____

_____

_____

_____

_____

_____

_____

Healing and the Mind

Health is not simply a medical term, it is a lifestyle choice—*choice* being the operative word here. Every thought, every emotion, and every attitude we choose to harbor has the ability to create health or compromise it.

> **The physics of happiness**
> - Life in the open air
> - Love for another being
> - Freedom from ambition
> - Creation
>
> *Albert Camus*—"The Four Conditions of Happiness"

And never ever forget that you are the choicemaker when it comes to your own personal feelings. Your feelings are yours, not someone else's, and not someone else's fault, either. No one is forcing you to feel anxiety when stuck in rush-hour traffic. No one is forcing you to feel guilt over how you treated an associate at work.

When you make the right lifestyle choices and experience true health you will feel a wholeness in body, mind, and spirit. These three components combined create your mindbody physiology.

When your mindbody physiology is in its most healthy state, you not only merge all the parts of yourself, but you also merge with the Earth's environment. You are able to realize that you are part of nature, not separate. You can see clearly that we are all made from recycled earth, water, and air—carbon, hydrogen, oxygen, nitrogen, and sulfur. We are made of the exact same stuff found in all of nature—the DNA configuration is the only difference. When we forget this and separate from Mother Nature, great dysfunction can result.

Just as Mother Earth has this incredible capacity to find homeostasis, or balance, so too can the human body. We live in a time, however, when we humans seem to be mindlessly compromising Mother Earth and disrupting her natural rhythms. This resonates in our bodies as well. When we repeatedly choose to ignore or live outside of the magnificent rhythms found in nature, we begin to feel the consequences.

Your Wellness Quotient

So what do you think about your most recent lifestyle choices? Let's step back and add all the elements of your existence together. This will give you your health profile, or wellness quotient.

As you consider recent attitudinal choices, do you see any recurring themes? Do you lack spirituality or a sense of purpose? Are you often pessimistic? Do you experience toxic relationships, skip meals, eat junk food, smoke, drink alcohol, take drugs, forgo exercise? If you answered "Yes" to any of my questions, then guess what . . . you exhibit a definite imbalance in your mindbody physiology, and you are putting yourself at high risk for some types of disease. A lack of connection with spirit—thus life-affirming lifestyle choices—over long periods of time can manifest as immune and nervous system malfunction, hormonal disturbances, heart disease, psychological problems, and, yes, possibly even cancer.

Don't worry. You can reverse harmful patterns by raising your consciousness, or getting in touch with spirit. When we live at a higher level of consciousness, we pay attention to our choices on several levels. Suddenly we not only know what we should eat, but also why we should eat these good things. We intuitively begin to know how and why physical activity is of the utmost importance for mindbody health. We begin to see why are we here and what we are meant to do with the precious gift of life. Please don't spend your time dying. Spend every moment living as fully and exultantly as you can.

Beauty and Wellness Integration

Beauty is health, and health becomes beauty. The two concepts create a mystical cycle, each fulfilling the other. There are many ways to integrate beauty and wellness into your professional services, and again, we come right back to attitude. Look at each beauty service as a wellness service. Whether performing a haircut, a facial, or a manicure, consider ways to expand your outlook—your perspective—until the line between beauty service and wellness service is not just blurred but gone!

- Bring yourself fully into the service.
- Create a glowing, healthy aura around the service.
- Deliver a pleasant and serene setting.
- Provide wonderful sights, from a fresh and clean station to flowers and all manner of beautiful color.
- Offer calming sounds, including music. Cut the noise pollution.
- Provide healing aromas.
- Engage all the senses with multipurpose and nurturing products.

In addition to how you approach your beauty services, you can also choose to offer clients specific beauty/wellness rituals. These services include aromatherapy, massage, acupuncture, herbal and flower essence therapies, Reiki (energy therapy), nutritional counseling, yoga, and meditation. All these feel-good practices, when combined with traditional beauty services, give clients a respite from their busy, stressful lives and encourage your clients' true inner and outer beauty to shine simultaneously.

As this book progresses, we will discuss some of these beauty practices in greater depth. For now, however, I want to explore two concepts that brilliantly integrate many of these beauty/wellness ceremonies. I am speaking of the chakra system and Ayurveda. Each represents a way of thinking, and each in its own unique way provides an overall outlook on life that gloriously produces ultimate health and beauty.

The Chakra System

Discovering and sharing the power of spiritual beauty can be accomplished in so many ways, but one path that has given me particularly profound insight is the chakra system. My hair professional performs a chakra-balancing haircut that is quite ritualistic and uses several different essential oils, flower essences, and plant oils in anointing the scalp, hair, neck, and shoulders. I feel like I've just taken a trip to the outermost regions of the cosmos after receiving this service. It is pure bliss! It is beauty and wellness integration at its best.

For those unfamiliar with the term *chakra*, it is a Sanskrit word that translates into *wheels of light*. This ancient Hindu concept relates to the seven energy centers found within each individual—the chakras. Each chakra, or center, is a vortex of energy, a spiritual opening in the body where subtle energies may enter and leave. Chakras process these energies and convert them into chemical, hormonal, and cellular changes in the body. The chakras act as doorways to our consciousness, allowing ethereal energy to become physical, and physical energy to return to the ethereal realm. It is in accessing energy through these doorways that our beliefs, emotions, and attitudes create our minds and bodies, and thus our reality. A positive state of well-being occurs when all the chakras are balanced.

Each chakra controls certain aspects of our spiritual, psychological, and physical development. Here is a brief overview of the seven major chakras.

1. *The Root or Base Chakra:* If you seek to balance the physical body, meditate on this chakra. Located at the base of the spine, it bestows the life force and is responsible for our feeling grounded and secure. It is also the seat of fear, particularly as related to our physical survival. This chakra controls our adrenals, kidneys, legs, feet, anus, and coccyx.

2. *The Navel or Hara Chakra:* If you want to release tension and allow your creativity to flow freely, meditate on this chakra. Located between the lower abdomen and navel, this chakra is responsible for the development of our sexuality, pleasure, and personal relationships. It controls the gonads, genitals, reproductive system, pelvis, belly, sacrum, and lumbar spine.

3. *The Solar Plexus Chakra:* If you have issues with your graciousness, self-confidence, or personal power, meditate on this chakra. Located above the navel and below the chest, it is responsible for self-control and the ability to manifest that which we desire. This chakra controls the pancreas, lumbar spine, stomach, gall bladder, liver, diaphragm, and nervous system.

4. *The Heart Chakra:* Meditate on this chakra to release feelings of love, joy, compassion, and peace. Located in the chest center, it concerns divine and unconditional love. All levels of love flow through this chakra, from self-love to cosmic love. As the seat of our soul, it governs our thymus, heart, circulatory system, lower lungs, chest, breasts, and thoracic spine.

5. *The Throat Chakra:* As you meditate on this chakra, release all thought and heed your inner voice of wisdom. Located in the throat area, it is responsible for self-expression, it bestows wisdom, and it gives us an ability to communicate our wisdom. This chakra affects the thyroid, throat, mouth, vocal cords, lungs, respiratory system, cervical spine, arms, and hands.

6. *The Third Eye or Brow Chakra:* Meditate on this chakra to awaken your spiritual vision and see all of creation with deep love. It gives us vision, concentration, and devotion to manifest dreams. Located in the center of the forehead, between the eyebrows, it bestows heightened intuition and clairvoyance. It controls our pituitary gland, nervous system, medulla cortex, base skull, forehead, nose, and left eye.

7. *The Crown Chakra:* Meditating on this chakra allows you to see your purest potentiality. Located at the top of the head, it bestows omnipotence and total freedom. This is where we see ourselves merging with universal spirit, experiencing divine consciousness and transcendence. This chakra controls the pineal gland, cranium, cerebral cortex, and right eye.

As you travel from the Root Chakra upward toward the Crown Chakra, vibrational frequency and intensity grow. Balancing the chakras can result in optimal vitality and health. It is through the chakra network that our body, mind, and spirit are woven together as one holistic system. Imbalances in any one of the chakras may show up as dysfunction or disease.

As spiritual beings, we strive to open all the chakras to their optimal energy flow and vibration, enabling ourselves to become harmonious, open channels to the universal spirit. Bringing a harmonious and balanced self into everything that we do becomes our gift to the world and our legacy when we leave this earthly plane.

Chakra-oriented services are now available in many salons and spas. Creative visualization, meditation, and energy work such as Reiki, massage, aura balancing, shiatsu, acupuncture, color therapy, and toning (using sound) are all ways in which alignment may be renewed within the chakra system.

Beauty Professional, Heal Thyself

As caregivers, it is essential that we take good care of ourselves. It is a vital first step toward giving our clients the best possible care. So as we delve into various spiritually oriented beauty and wellness techniques, I urge you to experience their magic for yourself first.

Before giving any service, take a moment to stabilize your energy and give it a boost. Sit quietly for a least a minute with eyes closed. Breathe deeply and smoothly. Visualize your feet grounded into the earth. See your energy merging with the Earth's energy. Feel the feedback loop. Feel the incredible pranic energy circuiting between you and the Earth. Gradually bring your attention back to your surroundings in the work environment. Gently open your eyes, enjoy a glass of pure water, perhaps a wholesome organic snack, and then proceed with your next service.

This solitary moment allows you to clear away any errant energy patterns that may be left over from the last service and greet the next service with present-moment awareness and utmost loving-kindness.

Making the Connection with Your Client

Before I give a body massage or begin a hair service, I place my hands on the client's scalp, or perhaps their shoulders, and speak gently to them. I breathe smoothly, deeply, and evenly as I am doing this.

Inevitably, my client begins to feel a calmness, tune in to me, and relax. A true connection between myself and my client takes place! This optimizes the ensuing experience for both giver and receiver. When I experience this in my work, I find meaning and higher purpose in what I do. See every moment spent in communion with another as an opportunity to bring centering and balance into your own life as well as those of others.

Give Your Clients a Hand

Reiki is fast becoming a standard offering in many holistic spas. Practitioners of this ancient Tibetan healing system use light hand placements to channel healing energies. While exact technique and philosophy may vary widely, Reiki is commonly used to treat emotional and mental distress as well as chronic and acute physical problems. It also assists the receiver in achieving spiritual focus and clarity.

What Are Flower Essences?

Flower essences are vibrational medicines, not to be confused with aromatherapy or essential oils. A flower essence is an odorless solution created by capturing the essence of a flower or plant through solar infusion in purified water. Known to aid the natural healing capacity of both the body and mind, the life force in flower essences resonate with and awaken particular qualities within the human soul. They work on every possible emotional level, from sensitivity to shame, creativity to prejudice, obsession to possessiveness. Flower essences are used to alleviate stressful emotional states that may hinder personal growth or may contribute to illness.

In the salon, you can serve beverages spiked with appropriate flower essences, then send the essence home with clients—after, of course, explaining the power of a flower essence! You can also empower shampoo and conditioning services or massage services by adding flower essences. You might try infusing flower essences into the air, choosing a different essence or a different combination of essences every day. Trust me, flower essences are a valuable therapy in these times, and the perfect fit for the spa or salon beauty and wellness environment. In addition to all the wonderfully healthful benefits you can give clients, adding flower essences to your retail inventory is a nice way to boost revenue.

Mindbody Health and Ayurveda

As mindbody health approaches go, Ayurveda is the great-great-great-great-grandmother of them all. Sanskrit for *the science of life*, Ayurveda is a medical science and system that has been practiced in India for over 5,000 years. At its heart and soul, Ayurveda guides us in recognizing that we *can* bring balance into our lives by making the correct lifestyle choices. Our most evolutionary choices can be achieved by tapping into a higher consciousness, and this most remarkable system teaches us to realize these choices through a variety of concepts, rituals, and practices, including sensory modulation techniques, meditation, Pranayama, and yoga.

Today Ayurveda is recognized by the World Health Organization as an effective health science, and it is currently undergoing extensive research at the U.S. National Institutes of Health. Many documented studies now suggest that Ayurvedic therapies may reduce cardiovascular disease risk factors (including blood pressure, cholesterol levels, and reaction to stress) as well as preventing or treating certain cancers, infectious diseases, immune system deficiencies, neurological disorders, and hormonal problems. More than a few champions of Ayurveda are also interested in its ability to slow the aging process.

The Natural Approach to Health

Ayurveda and mindbody health are intrinsically linked. I adhere to Ayurvedic practices in my life because they honor the most simple and natural of approaches toward balance and well-being. These natural therapies include meditation, yoga, all forms of physical activity, Pranayama (breathing practices), regular connection with nature, nutrition, herbal therapies, and sensory modulation techniques such as massage, aroma, color, and sound/music therapies.

Ayurveda focuses on the nature of the mindbody connection—the balance between mind, body, and spirit. Ayurveda teaches that every experience we have—including our perceptions, interpretations, and lifestyle choices—is metabolized into molecules within our bodies. Therefore, it can be said that our bodies and the ways in which we perceive our world are a direct result of what we experience in our consciousness.

Through this time-honored science of life, each one of us recognizes our uniqueness. Each one of us has our own constitution and temperament, a mindbody network that influences our physical appearance along with the way we typically think, react, eat, and sleep.

Begin at the Beginning

Ayurvedic treatment challenges us to bring natural balance into our lives through the choices that we make. While some of these choices can be quite soulful, many are as simple as creating a daily routine that promotes stability. Stability is a wonderful, soothing mechanism when everything else is chaotic. It gives you time and space to connect with mind, body, and spirit. Happily, this first step toward mindfulness doesn't come in a bottle, is accessible to everyone, and costs nothing. Here are a few ways to create stability and thus mindfulness in your life:

- Go to bed early and rise early.
- Take time for reflection, meditation, and breathing practices.
- See all physical activity as consciousness in motion.
- Eat simple, pure, whole, organic foods and prepare these meals with a joyous and loving spirit.
- Minimize disturbing influences.
- Enjoy every facet of nature, as often as you can.
- SLOW DOWN and enjoy every bullet point above!

Take a few moments to jot down ways in which you might change your daily routine in order to promote stability in your life.

_____

_____

_____

_____

_____

_____

_____

_____

_____

_____

_____

Mindfulness

THE QUESTIONER: What is it that you and your disciples practice?

BUDDHA: We sit, we walk, and we eat.

THE QUESTIONER: Doesn't everyone sit, walk, and eat?

BUDDHA: Yes, but when we sit we know we are sitting. When we walk we know we are walking, and when we eat we know we are eating.

In this we find the essence of mindfulness, which means simply paying attention to the moment. You become intimately connected to an actual moment—from obvious occurrences to subtle nuances. If connected to this moment right now, you should be able to see yourself reading these words, see yourself reflecting on their meaning, see yourself reacting to the meaning. You are in essence communing with your higher self, and mindful of all that is happening.

Make every moment of every day a celebration of mindfulness. Instead of jumping out of bed when the alarm blares, give yourself time to relish the early morning light and sounds. Do deep breathing and gentle stretching exercises while still in bed. As the day progresses, remain mindful of all you do, whether washing dishes, brushing your teeth, eating dinner, making love, cutting a head of hair, or giving a massage.

Write down a few of your routine daily activities. Celebrate them. Become mindful and witness them. What is it about brushing your teeth that makes today's effort different from yesterday's?

_____

_____

_____

_____

_____

_____

_____

_____

_____

_____

_____

_____

The Science of Life

Ayurveda recognizes that five great elements create the universe, which includes us. These elements are referred to as space, air, fire, earth, and water. Inherent in all of creation, these elements combine with each other to create three mindbody principles or doshas. There is the Air or Vata dosha, the Fire or Pitta dosha, and the Earth or Kapha dosha.

These mindbody principles relate to the cosmic rhythms—circadian, seasonal, lunar, and tidal—and the principles will ebb and flow according to changes in the cosmic rhythms as well as in our temperaments and body health.

Throughout nature, there are never-ending cycles of communication, transformation, regeneration, and reproduction. These cycles affect singular cells as well as complex organisms. In respecting the cosmic rhythms instead of thwarting them, we encourage the effortless flow of intelligence through our bodies. We also safeguard the natural order of our bodily functions, including our sleep/wake cycle, body temperature, hormonal output and fluctuation, regenerative capabilities, metabolism, and reproductive cycles. In other words, there is an optimal time in the course of every 24-hour circadian cycle for waking, sleeping, eating, physical activity, and heightened creativity, as well as for the elimination of toxins. We only need to tune in to the rhythms of nature as well as to our personal sensations and intuitions.

If you work every night until 10 P.M. and regularly go out after work for dinner or socializing, you are up and about when you are meant to be getting valuable shut-eye and regenerating your body. Working the night shift, gambling through the night in a Las Vegas casino, making a transcontinental flight, or eating a large meal before bed: these are all additional ways we can throw off our biological rhythms. When these rhythms are consistently thwarted and go out of whack, dysfunction may result.

What can we do? Well, we can work toward honoring the natural order of things and work toward moderation. Check abhorrent behavior at the door, before it gets the better of you! Work toward detoxifying and revitalizing the natural world. Remember, pollution begins in the mind.

The Rhythms of Nature

The universe is constantly playing an incredible symphony. Everything happens in rhythm. The seasons, the beating of a heart, day and night, the coming and going of migratory birds, flowers that wake up and then sleep, it's all part of life's tempo. When I speak of tuning in, it is truly about feeling the pulse of the planet and sensing nature's rhythms. You can feel and see the earth breathe. You will hear it humming.

The Mindbody Principles

Ayurveda theory states that all humans come ready-made with three inherent mindbody principles—air, fire, and earth—and an energy is associated with each of these principles. Each person has one or two dominant energies, but all three need to be balanced in order to find true and complete inner beauty.

That Which Moves Things—The Air mindbody principle or air energy represents movement, including movement of the body, blood, food, and thoughts. Air is light, cold, dry, irregular, and highly active. Those with a predominant Air mindbody principle are naturally lively and stimulating. To protect their mindbody physiology and maintain balance, these individuals should go the extra mile when it comes to getting ample sleep, eating a regular and healthful diet, and avoiding that which brings anxiety.

That Which Digests Things—The Fire mindbody principle or fire energy represents chemical transformation and light. Fire is hot, intense, penetrating, pungent, and illuminating. Think metabolism. It helps modulate our ability to digest—including food, emotions, and ideas. Individuals with a predominant Fire principle are known for their sharp intellect, strong passion, and highly focused ambition. An unbalanced Fire principle can result in chronic heartburn, uncontrollable temper tantrums, and other maladies.

That Which Holds Things Together—The Earth mindbody principle or earth energy represents structure, stability, and lubrication. Earth is cold, heavy, stable, slow, and cohesive. It helps modulate the building of tissues, organs, and bones. It can also optimize fluids in the body and the environment. Anyone with a predominant Earth principle should remain true to his or her down-to-earth and easygoing self. When the Earth energy is unbalanced, one may suffer lethargy, depression, and physical congestion.

What Is Your Energy?

The following questionnaire was developed by David Simon, M.D., Medical Director and Co-Founder of the Chopra Center for Well Being in La Jolla, California, www.chopra.com. It offers an excellent starting point to determine your primary mindbody energy according to Ayurveda theory. In each category, place a check under the one or two statements that best describe your physical characteristics. At the end, add up the check marks in each column. The higher total(s) denote a dominance of this dosha.

For a more in-depth assessment of your doshic energies, consider a seminar and/or workshop available through the Chopra Center for Well Being. (See resources section in this book.)

Physical Characteristic	Vata (Air)	Pitta (Fire)	Kapha (Earth)
Frame	○ I am slender with prominent joints and thin muscles.	○ I have a medium, symmetrical build with good muscle development.	○ I have a large, stocky build. My frame is broad, stout or thick.
Weight	○ Low; I may forget to eat or have a tendency to lose weight.	○ Moderate; it is easy for me to gain or lose weight if I put my mind to it.	○ Heavy; I gain weight easily and have difficulty losing it.
Eyes	○ I have average or small eyes.	○ I tend to have an intense gaze.	○ I have large pleasant eyes.
Complexion	○ My skin tends to be dry or thin.	○ My skin is warm, reddish in color and prone to irritation.	○ My skin is thick, moist, and smooth.
Hair	○ My hair tends to be dry or frizzy.	○ My hair is fine with a tendency towards early thinning or graying.	○ I have abundant, thick and oily hair.
Joints	○ My joints are thin and prominent, and have a tendency to crack.	○ My joints are loose and flexible.	○ My joints are large, well knit and padded.
Sleep Pattern	○ I am a light sleeper with a tendency to awaken easily.	○ I am a moderately sound sleeper, usually needing less than eight hours to feel rested.	○ My sleep is deep and long. I tend to awaken slowly in the morning.
Body Temperature	○ My hands and feet are usually cold and I prefer warm environments.	○ I am usually warm, regardless of the season, and prefer cooler environments.	○ I am adaptable to most temperatures but do not like cold, wet days.
Temperament	○ I am lively and enthusiastic by nature. I like to change.	○ I am purposeful and intense. I like to convince.	○ I am easy going and accepting. I like to support.
Under Stress . . .	○ I become anxious and/or worried.	○ I become irritable and/or aggressive.	○ I become withdrawn and/or reclusive.
TOTALS	Vata _____	Pitta _____	Kapha _____

Balance Your Energy

All three mindbody principles or energies are in us and around us, although each one of us usually has one predominant energy. When in balance, these energies are magnificent to behold and bring into our lives all the very best. If, however, your dominant energy becomes unbalanced, problems may arise.

If you've ever been tempted to call someone an airhead, this person is probably ruled by the air energy, and it's out of balance. They perhaps have too much movement or irregularity in their lives. They may need to bring calming practices into their life that will ground them and bring them back down to earth.

How about the time you called someone a hothead? This person's fire energy is most likely unbalanced. The chemical transformation and light in this individual may be too intense. Out-of-balance fire energies need to be pacified by cooling them.

Unbalanced earth energy tends to make one heavy and too grounded—with lethargy, indecisiveness, and complacency as possible results. This person has likely taken on too much structure or weight. The result? "Couch potato" comes to mind! Out-of-balance earth energy needs stimulation to get the mindbody physiology moving.

By tapping into our energetic natures, we open the door to our consciousness and learn so much about ourselves. We begin to understand why we enjoy certain activities and dread others. We discover why we react in certain ways to one situation and completely differently to another. For example, a person governed by the air principle tends to feel cold more often than not, and thus will enjoy traveling to a sultry, warm climate. A predominant fire type will be more drawn to ski vacations in the Rocky Mountains. An earth type may lament that they can just look at a piece of chocolate cake and put on weight, while the typically slim air type can often eat anything without gaining weight.

In addition to the fascinating things Ayurveda teaches us about ourselves, a keen understanding of human energy patterns may help you deal more productively with others. You may find yourself feeling more compassion or empathy for a feisty client or fussy guest—because the "why" behind the feistiness or fussiness is suddenly apparent.

What we've covered here only brushes the surface of Ayurveda theory. If you want to learn more, many wonderful books and educational programs explain these concepts further.

Directed Energy

Many spas today feature Ayurvedic therapies, particularly in hair and skin care. Beyond the general goodness that these services bring to clients, Ayurveda practices can also be used to address specific beauty problems. Dry skin is generally an air imbalance; premature graying or hair thinning can be attributed to a fire imbalance; excessively oily skin may be attributed to earth energy gone awry.

If you are interested in these beauty-directed Ayurvedic concepts, there are books, seminars, and entire product lines popping up. Check them out!

A Wellness Culture

Everything we've discussed so far should give you a better picture of how your inner environment promotes spiritual beauty. In addition to the services you provide, the information you share, and the attitudes you prescribe to, the outer environment in which you work also affects your connection to spiritual beauty.

Turn your spa or salon into a space where the environment and everyone in it is permeated by holistic thoughts, actions, conversations, sights, sounds, and smells. And yes, an environment does have its own energy. It is a living, breathing, metabolizing, conscious entity. The lighting, colors, aromas, and sounds all send different expressions of energy, and these can all have tremendous impact on the sense of wellness that radiates from your workplace environment.

The Spa/Salon Spiritualized

It is so important to honor the multidimensional layers of our work environment. The more spiritually sustaining your workplace is, the happier and healthier you will be. In addition, when you feel supported and cared for within the working environment, you are more able to nurture your customers.

Any of the following ideas help turn the beauty environment into a spiritually satisfying place—an environment where beauty and wellness become deeply integrated. While each suggestion is designed to serve you, the beauty professional, you'll immediately see how several benefit clients as well.

- Serve healthful beverages instead of the typical soda and coffee. Think organic tea, coffee (with organic cream and sugar!), juices, or purified water.
- Have fresh fruit available.
- Always take a lunch break. Your physical as well as emotional health depends on it.
- Connect with nature—it is a prime source for spiritual sustenance. Take a break, go outside, walk around, and breathe deeply.
- Make sure your work environment includes some or all of the following: natural light, skylights, full-spectrum lighting fixtures, green (real) plants, waterfalls, natural and sustainable materials (i.e. recycled wood, cork, bamboo, recycled glass, marble).
- Encourage recycling in your work environment. If you and your fellow beauty pros are not already doing this, find out why not! Lead an effort to make this happen. We must refashion, renew, revive, revolve, reuse, and recycle as much as possible.
- If possible, create a small ritual place outside the salon or spa for staff or vendor meetings. These types of nature breaks can greatly revive, refresh, and renew the spirit. Your place need not be a huge deal. A few chairs beside a simple, decorative bench or bistro table, just outside the front door and surrounded with potted plants, will work wonderfully.
- Encourage regular company get-togethers, such as picnics, backyard barbecues, or retreats. Make acknowledgment of achievements and milestones, and expression of gratitude and lovingkindness part of these gatherings.
- As part of each day, engage in some form of healthful exercise, such as stretching, yoga, or walking. Form an early-morning walking or yoga club. Invite a yoga instructor into the salon. Request that the instructor concentrate on ways to enjoy short yoga breaks throughout the day.
- Honor creative expression in the workplace by displaying employees' poetry, paintings, sculpture, and craftwork.
- Create and display a company vision statement, stressing the importance of mutual respect and trust amongst the team of beauty professionals within this environment.
- Make sure that everyone tries every service offered by your company. This allows each person to feel a part of the team and also confident in recommending a service to a client.

- Encourage intellectual stimulation and spiritual growth through continuing education. Along with more traditional beauty or business fare, consider a book club, book readings, or poetry slams, as well as in-house instructional seminars on meditation, yoga, nutrition, stress reduction, and other wellness practices.

Consider gathering with fellow beauty professionals to discuss wellness and spiritual issues. These meetings can take place in the work environment or at an off-site location. If you are in the employ of another, secure this person's permission first and be sure to include him or her in your gathering!

During your meetings, use a circle process, in which each voice is heard. Paramount to the success of your circle gathering is total trust in the group, along with the ability to listen. This process has been around for over 60,000 years. See your circle as a community of like-minded individuals working toward implementing their values as a group. Discuss anything you would like to see changed in the workplace environment, anything you feel is working, and any possible new processes. Have someone take minutes and put these notes in a binder for all to reference as needed—and perhaps this may even spawn a newsletter or content for a salon/spa web site.

Besides sharing ideas, you can also invite in experts to teach new ideas. You can collectively smudge the salon or spa and meeting room (see page 65 for smudge definition), or your circle group can share a splendidly peaceful moment of Pranayama and yoga.

People I would like to invite to a beauty and wellness gathering:

_____

_____

_____

_____

_____

_____

Subjects our gathering might explore (and the appropriate experts to teach them):

_____

_____

_____

_____

_____

_____

_____

Write down at least five ways you could create a more spiritual environment in your workplace. Think about these practices and concepts as they relate to yourself individually, within your own small sphere of influence. Then think more broadly, expanding your view outward to the environment as a whole. Once you complete these five concepts, try coming up with five more. In time, you will find yourself spending each working day in a most wonderful, nurturing environment. Don't be surprised if neither you nor your clients ever want to leave!

_____

_____

_____

_____

_____

_____

_____

_____

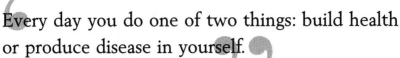

> Every day you do one of two things: build health or produce disease in yourself.
>
> *Adelle Davis*

Smudge Your Environment

The Native American practice of smudging represents a sacred ritual in which loose or bundled aromatic herbs (sage, cedar, copal, yerba santa, and juniper, to name a few) are burned in order to bring in blessings and purification and smoke out negative energies. The herbs are lit over a ceramic bowl, or smudge pot, and the embers are gently blown to create smoke. The smoke may be used to purify the body, the home, the salon or spa, or any gathering, healing, or meditation space.

Consider smudging the salon or spa in the morning before clients arrive. It's all about surrounding yourself and your environment with a higher vibrational frequency.

The Top Ten Youthing Practices/Techniques

Remember, you are a choicemaker. Every day you elect to either nurture health and beauty or deplete them. Choose the former and I guarantee you will soon begin to feel a renewed youthfulness and vitality. Here are a few of my favorite primary techniques or practices that can help you feel youthful, regardless of your literal age.

1. Reduce stress and see with clarity your purpose in life. Meditate, pray, practice deep breathing, creative visualization, and positive affirmations. These approaches help reduce detrimental effects of stress while also raising your level of mindfulness and honing your intuitive instincts.
2. Maximize your nutrition to optimize your energy. Eat an organic, whole-foods diet. Take in nourishment with full awareness.
3. Keep your body hydrated to enhance a wide range of metabolic functions. Water is responsible for oxygenating your blood while also providing an additional energy source. For maximum benefit, drink one quart for every 50 pounds of body weight.
4. Stay physically active to create energy. Build extra movement into every moment of every day. Consider a balance of activities that will benefit cardiovascular functioning, flexibility, and strength.

> "You're never too old to become younger."
>
> *Mae West*

5. Get adequate rest so the body's regenerative processes can proceed as you sleep. Sleep deprivation can zap mental energy, disrupt normal body functions (hormone levels, heart rate, blood pressure, and body temperature), and block creative energy. It can also wreak havoc with your body's seratonin levels, which can consequently effect your feelings of well-being and happiness.

6. Indulge in massage to de-stress and energize your body and rid it of toxins, and to alleviate some forms of pain. When our skin is stroked, a flood of feel-good chemicals is released into the blood stream, including natural antidepressants, natural Valium, and natural growth hormones.

7. Practice good skin care for inner and outer beauty. The primary function of the skin—the body's largest organ—is to help the body eliminate toxins through perspiration. To keep this remarkable system up and running, cleanse, moisturize, detoxify, exfoliate, and protect through a regular and organic skin-care regimen.

8. Good elimination rids toxins from the system. Include plenty of fiber in your diet (25–35 grams a day), drink at least eight 8-ounce glasses of water a day (not iced!), get regular aerobic exercise to tone the intestinal muscles, and consume live active cultures like those found in yogurt, kefir, or high-quality probiotic supplements.

9. Give yourself miles of smiles. When you smile, you rev up the immune system, lower blood pressure, and promote better sleep as well as several other beneficial physiological changes.

10. Establish a daily routine that promotes inner and outer balance. If possible, go to bed and wake up at the same time every day. Take nourishment at regular times. Follow holistic beautifying rituals. Honor yourself by trying not to take on more than you can handle. Connect with nature daily. Practice moderation in everything.

Many of you may have your own versions of these techniques. That's okay. Do whatever feels right, as long as these techniques bring you to your optimum state of beauty and wellness. Remember, physical health and well-being means the absence of disease and also the presence of joy, vitality, energy, alertness, creativity, confidence, and love.

Notes:

Chapter Four

Life's Great Balancing Act

> For years, the American dream was epitomized by more, bigger, better, and faster. No longer. Quality of life is more important. One thing you can be sure of is that masses of us are looking for a slice of life that's easier, happier, and more straightforward, a return to a simple, honest life.
>
> *Faith Popcorn*

Futurists like Alvin Toffler, author of such notable books as *Future Shock*, propose that 95 percent of everything that's been discovered or invented in the entire history of the world was discovered or invented in the twentieth century. In fact, some say that our bodies and minds are so acclimated to change that now we can speed up, but we can't slow down. Futurist Edie Weiner suggests this: if we woke up twenty-five years in the future, we could probably acclimate ourselves within a month. If we woke up twenty-five years in the past, we wouldn't be able to survive.

As we career into the twenty-first century, change continues in overdrive. Many of these changes are considered progress. Some are considered downright regression. Still others are viewed as improvements, but with a price, for even the most widely acclaimed progress may bring deep-rooted insecurities due to globalization and political and sociocultural influences. There's no place to hide from these influences, since the media feeds us a daily diet of worldwide disaster. Violence, famine, disease, natural and manmade catastrophes—they all ride on the coattails of change. This constant exposure to life's frailties can cause overwhelming stress.

I feel it is vital that we humans take any and every step possible to create inner balance. It is more important than ever that we dedicate some portion of our time to stress relief and simplification. We must create symmetry or balance between "giddy-up go" and "Whoa! "Too many of us have forgotten how to enjoy life. As Albert Einstein said, "It has become appallingly obvious that our technology has exceeded our humanity."

Identifying Different Stressors

Many healers today ascribe to a belief that we humans are disconnected from our deepest, truest selves, distracted and overwhelmed by the speed of life. Everywhere we turn, someone or something is telling us how we should look, act, and be. We're dancing as fast as we can to accommodate society's standards. Consequently we're losing our balance and tripping over every little fad. Sadly, as we lose contact with our inner selves, we create a breeding ground for stress—or should I say *dis*tress? It is essential to identify and eliminate (or at least reduce) the sources of these negative mental stressors.

As if this isn't enough, we humans suffer additional emotional stress from toxic relationships and the toxic byproducts generated by these detrimental relationships.

All these emotional stressors wreak havoc on our biological systems, leading to fatigue, life-threatening disease, and everything in between.

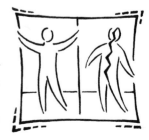

Along with emotional stress, we expose ourselves every day to environmental stressors. I refer to life-threatening toxins in the food we eat, the air we breathe, and the water we drink.

> **You** ask me how I can remain calm and not become upset when those around me are all bustling about. What can I say to you? I did not come into the world to agitate it. Is it not sufficiently agitated already?
>
> *St. Francois de Sales*

Environmental pollution diminishes our energy while also disturbing our natural filtration and digestive systems.

Indeed, we live in stressful times, and it has never been more important to simplify our lives, realize what is truly important, and listen to our inner voice—our spirit. When you awaken to spirit, it becomes much easier to develop coping mechanisms.

In this chapter we will first define and identify different stressors in life. Then we will explore practices to reduce or manage these different stressors. In particular we will discuss the enormous benefits of breathwork and meditation. Use these destressing techniques along with those previously covered, including positive affirmations, creative visualization, attitude adjustment, emotional clearing, and the development of compassion. Lest you think I'm ignoring the importance of nutrition, physical activity, and sensory modulation when it comes to stress management, rest easy. Succeeding chapters will cover these three very important approaches to mindbody health.

What Exactly Is Stress?

Stress, as explained by the Wellness Councils of America, is *the inability to cope with a threat, real or imagined, to our well-being, which results in a series of responses and adaptations by our minds and bodies.* The World Health Organization claims that stress is now officially a worldwide epidemic.

The Stress Response

When we experience stress, our adrenal glands pump adrenaline into the bloodstream. As the adrenaline surges through our bodies, it gives us an energy boost to fight or take flight from the perceived stressor. A manageable amount of stress, called *eustress*, is actually a good thing, required by all humans in order to maintain optimal health and continued growth. When stress is perceived by the mindbody physiology as excessive, however, *distress* results.

Perhaps you've heard the story about the grandmother who lifted a car off someone trapped underneath. This is the fight-or-flight response in action, with "fight" winning out. Manageable stress can give us uncommon strength and fortitude to face a challenge or perceived threat. If one does not have the coping mechanism to calm down after this initial response to stress, or if stress is being experienced on a constant basis, then the adrenal cortex begins to secrete detrimental hormones into the system. If bad stress hormones are allowed to hum along unabated, then potentially debilitating or life-threatening consequences can result. You could end up compromising your immune system, as well as causing adrenal exhaustion, high blood pressure, heart disease, cancer, and diabetes. It is absolutely essential to identify bad stressors and learn how to counter them.

Stress and Free Radicals

Among other things, stress forms free radicals in the body. Free radical formation, or oxidation, is at the core of aging and at the root of more than sixty major illnesses, including heart disease, stroke, cancer, and cataracts. Some amount of free radical formation is natural, produced through cell metabolism. Stress—emotional, biological, and environmental—produces free-radical levels beyond what our bodies can handle, and thus has a connection to disease.

Free radicals occur when atoms break down and, in the process, lose electrons. These atoms steal electrons from neighboring atoms, setting up a cascading effect of electron thievery and a general breakdown of our molecules, cells, and tissues. What I've just described is an accelerated aging process. As free-radical formation accelerates, so does the aging process.

To prevent or stave off the detrimental effects of free radicals, you want to first and foremost clear unmanageable stress out of your life. At the very least, reduce it until it's manageable. Meditation coupled with Pranayama—healthful breathing practices—are excellent practices to help shift your perceptions of and attitude toward stress. You also want to get an ample supply of antioxidants every day. You'll find plenty of antioxidants in organic, whole foods such as fresh fruits and vegetables. You can also fortify your diet with a high-quality multivitamin and antioxidant supplements, namely vitamins C, E, B_6, beta carotene, selenium, and CoQ_{10} enzyme.

> *All things are living, all things are dancing in the rhythm of eternal harmony.*
>
> Paramahansa Yogananda

Naturally, mindful physical activity goes the distance when it comes to effective stress reduction measures.

Environmental Stress

In physics, "organic" essentially means living. All things in our universe—including ourselves—that appear to exist independently are actually part of one all-encompassing organic pattern, and no one part of this pattern is separate from another. Nature functions as a living, breathing, metabolizing, conscious organism. When all parts hum along in harmony, true health, beauty, and balance result.

Mother Earth, as well as our bodies, has this incredible built-in healing system that maintains homeostasis—an ability to preserve internal equilibrium by adjusting physiological processes. This is part of the miracle we call life.

The ability to maintain organic stability even when natural conditions are disrupted is today being seriously challenged. An overwhelming amount of toxic chemical exposure experienced in our daily lives is creating an imbalance in nature and causing great stress. There are over 75,000 synthetic chemicals percolating throughout our environment. On a good day, we have about 400 toxic chemicals coursing through our veins.

Living an organic life is a conscious choice that greatly reduces many of these environmental stressors. Living organically is aligned with deeply held philosophical beliefs that serve to protect and nurture Mother Earth and in turn ourselves. Nature has been evolving for billions of years, and we should strive to understand and encourage conservation of her natural systems. As citizens of this planet, we must remember our place within and around these systems. There is just no good reason to level a rain forest, poison a lake, or contaminate a field with toxic materials.

Hopefully the salon or spa where you work is earth friendly! You all recycle. You try to reduce consumption. Products are holistic and certified organic. The environment is built from as many natural, sustainable materials as possible. Cleaning products are nontoxic. Clothing, towels, and sheets are organic. Food and beverages for staff and clients alike are nutritious and preferably organic. Water is purified. Reduce, reuse, recycle, rethink, and make all good choices for yourself, your clients, and our dear planet Earth. If these qualities are missing from your work environment, perhaps you can provide the initiative for change.

Organic Energy and Matter

What does "organic" mean, you ask? Some define organic plants as those grown in harmony with the natural rhythms of the universe. Others define "organic" as grown without use of toxic pesticides or nitrate-laden fertilizers. Both meanings are correct. On the broadest level, it is about a holistic thought process, an understanding that the life-force energy flowing through you and me is the same life-force energy flowing through Mother Earth. Anything we do to impact this beautiful flow of life-force energy has the potential to bring on an imbalanced state, a state that can, over time, create an accumulation of disease-related toxins. I urge you to live as organically as possible. This should be a conscious choice, a desire to dramatically limit exposure to toxic chemicals in food, beverages, and products. This includes cleaning products, personal care items, and garden products. And as organic thought processes go, it refers to the loving and holistic thoughts that you flow outward to all of creation. I cannot stress enough that organicism is not only about the products we use, but also the loving thoughts we generate.

The Spa/Salon Environment: A Sensory Experience

A salon or spa can be a potentially toxic environment. I am referring to environmental stressors such as toxic building materials, inadequate ventilation, temperature extremes, contact with harmful products, unhealthy fragrance molecules, and deficient or harsh lighting, as well as toxic noise levels. Even the layout of your workspace can cause environmental stress.

Many holistic salon owners across the United States make it their goal to create an environment that is energizing and devoid of as many potential environmental stressors as possible. Everything that goes into a building is being rethought, in order to reduce or eliminate such things as volatile organic compounds in wall paint, carpeting, or vinyl floor covering, and toxic chemicals in salon or spa products. Beauty professionals and clients are unanimously welcoming these environmentally stress-free surroundings, and this concept probably represents our profession's next wave of progress. With an enormous increase in allergies, asthma, and general negative reactions to synthetic environments (what the medical profession calls Multiple Chemical Sensitivities Disorder), there is no way it is *not* going to happen.

What Chemicals?

Even minor chemical exposures can add up when you consider the thousands of common and not-so-common chemicals that we experience every day. Answer the following questions to see how chemically laden your environment is. Don't be surprised if you're surprised!

1. Do you shampoo and condition your hair every morning?
2. Do you shower in chlorinated water?
3. Do you dress in clothing made from synthetic fiber?
4. Do you ride to work in a car or on a bus?
5. Do you work in an environment without adequate ventilation or operating windows?
6. Do you have consistent contact with chemical-laden products at work?
7. Do you work all day surrounded by fragrances?
8. Is there carpeting or vinyl flooring in your workspace?
9. Do you cook on a gas stove?
10. Do you eat processed foods, wrapped in plastic and made from conventionally produced plants or conventionally raised animals?
11. Do you sleep on non-organic sheets or a latex mattress?
12. Do you walk through and inhale in the detergent aisle at your local grocery store?
13. Do you walk across grass treated with lawn chemicals?

Did you do any or all of these things today? Everything mentioned here does have a natural, non-toxic alternative, and choosing any one of these alternatives can help de-stress your environment!

Research the Products You Use

If you have concerns about chemicals in any of the products used at work, do some research. Begin by asking the product manufacturer, representative, or educator about what's in their product and checking out any potential allergic reactions. Ask to see the Material Safety Data Sheets (MSDS) for any questionable products. They list product ingredients along with potential toxicities, storage requirements, product longevity, and safety/first aid guidelines. The salon or spa where you work should have them available; if not, request that they be obtained. The Occupational Safety and Health Administration (OSHA) requires that they be made available upon request. For more in-depth research related to cosmetic ingredients, I highly recommend that you turn to Ruth Winter's *A Consumer Dictionary of Cosmetic Ingredients* (fifth edition).

Green Your Indoor Air

Don't forget our potted plant friends. Some plants scrub the air of toxins while also keeping it humidified. Scatter organic greenery around your house and throughout your workspace. There is a wonderful book on this subject by B. C. Wolverton (Penguin Books) called *How to Grow Fresh Air: Fifty Houseplants that Purify Your Home and Office.* Some examples: The spider plant and the golden pothos both remove carbon monoxide as well as formaldehyde. English Ivy and the peace lily remove benzene. The potted mum and peace lily remove trichloroethylene. These living air filters have yet another benefit—color! Green is the color of the heart chakra, and this color is considered very cleansing as well as balancing for all matters of the heart.

Protect Your Skin

Beauty professionals routinely put their skin in jeopardy by handling toxic chemicals found in common hair and beauty products. The skin is living, breathing tissue; it can absorb chemicals, and it will allow chemicals to enter the bloodstream. Case in point: the large variety of dermal patches being used today to administer medicine.

Protect your skin. Become informed about the products you work with. Wear gloves whenever possible. Apply hydrating, emollient skin cream throughout the day. If you're about to cut a damp head of hair, rub leave-in hair conditioner into your hands before beginning—good for your hands and the client's hair! Select holistic products. It's all about raising your consciousness in the vitally important area of intelligent choice-making.

Environmental Stress Evaluation

It's a good idea to conduct a wellness audit in your work environment. (Consider auditing your home environment as well!) Evaluate the following and make (or suggest to your team leader) any necessary de-stressing alterations.

- *Ventilation*—Preferably you have extraction ventilation systems in your work environment, thus ensuring an ongoing supply of fresh air throughout the day.
- *Lighting*—Full-spectrum lighting is best, since it most closely simulates natural daylight. Colors will be truer and fatigue will be lessened.
- *Sound*—Decibel levels should be mindfully kept at a minimum to prevent toxic amounts of noise.
- *EMFs*—All electrical appliances put out electromagnetic frequencies (EMFs). Ever since the National Institute of Environmental Health Sciences labeled EMFs as a possible carcinogen, several manufacturers have introduced products with greatly reduced EMF levels. Be aware!
- *Nutritional sustenance*—Serving healthy food and beverages to yourself as well as your clients is imperative.
- *Sanitation*—How does your work environment measure up? Make sure you take full responsibility for and participate in healthy sanitation measures.
- *Industrial Safety Issues (OSHA)*—Become aware of regulations as they apply to your work environment, whether relative to sanitation, product, or safety issues.

(This evaluation is taken from one part of the Health Risk Appraisal (HRA) from the Wellness Councils of America. See the resource section for more information.)

Modern Life and Stress

In addition to environmental stressors, we also suffer from emotional stressors—unless you live in a Himalayan cave, this second category of stress is a fact of life. Our lifestyle largely determines these stressors, which may include work-family conflicts, financial pressures, work pressures, and simply feeling as if there's never enough time. Inadequate nutrition is also an indirect emotional stressor. A poor diet can make you feel tired, edgy, or irritable, and thus less able to respond rationally to any given negative situation. Uncontrolled stress creates a major risk factor for disease, but if you command healthy coping mechanisms and, most importantly, have mastered optimism and resiliency, you can combat these emotionally draining stressors.

To begin with, you must realize that your perception of a situation often exacerbates emotional stress. We've already discussed how important it is to change your thoughts, emotions, and beliefs if you feel that they are counterproductive to achieving your highest good. Making these positive changes may be the best coping mechanism of all. Positive thoughts, healthy emotions, and nurturing beliefs can dramatically shift stress responses in your body and lessen or stop the flow of detrimental stress hormones into your system. To realize these de-stressing changes, I strongly suggest that you routinely practice deep breathing exercises as well as imaging or visualizing desirable circumstances. Don't forget to do some emotional cleansing as well. You *can* change a mind-set that perceives work or home situations as threatening.

I could probably write an entire book about the stressors that plant themselves firmly in front of us each day. I think every one of us has different perceptions and descriptions of that which we find stressful. What I find compelling is how one person's stress is another person's glory. Some of us may break out in a cold sweat when we think about white-water rafting, parachuting, or trying some super-duper roller coaster. For others, however, these experiences are pure exhilaration and fun. Divorce may throw one person into utter despair and depression, while another feels unbridled freedom. One beauty professional might perceive a packed-solid appointment book as the epitome of efficiency, flowing creativity, and success, while another reacts by going into full-tilt panic. Every one of us reacts to stress in our own way. Every one of us also has the power to manage and reduce stress, change our perception of stressful experiences, and get the upper hand.

Stress in the Workplace

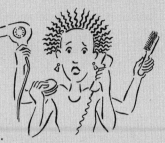

We've discussed how the quality of service you provide is a direct reflection of your attitude and your quality of life—two elements that contribute hugely to your state of health. And your state of health is intrinsically linked to how you handle stress.

Undeniably, as a beauty professional, you administer to a variety of client needs. No matter how much of this nurturing comes from the heart, it still remains a fact that all this caregiving can exacerbate emotional stress.

Read through the following situations and reflect on what your response or course of action might be. Make this an exercise in observing your reactions and then learning how to modulate your thoughts for ultimate peace of mind and well-being. Remember that every thought we have creates a molecular reaction in the body.

- You arrive at the salon after rushing to get there on time and hear that your first appointment canceled.
- You are booked every half-hour for eight consecutive hours— without one break.
- The front desk refuses to lower the music level despite repeated requests from you as well as from clients.
- Your client is unhappy with her finished cut and color. She creates a scene in the salon.
- You're partway through a facial service when you realize that you're really not there with the client. Your attention and energy has been focused on the yet-unresolved fight you had with your spouse last night.
- You've been working hard all day, receiving and serving clients, each one with personal needs and desires. You now feel absolutely zapped of energy. That breakfast yogurt and cup of coffee have long since cycled through your system.

- You're not sure how you're going to pay your rent this month. Business has been slow, and you're anticipating yet another small paycheck this week.
- You've been standing all day, your "dogs" are howling, and a dull ache throbs in your lower back. You are having a difficult time communicating with the client in your chair because all you can think about is getting off work.
- One of your associates grabs every possible opportunity to criticize your work, your dress, and anything else concerning you!

How did you do on this exercise? Did you answer more than one with an angry or perhaps dejected response? Next time you find yourself in any of these situations, use good old common sense and follow your gut instinct. You can come up with beneficial and healthful answers! Your own inner wisdom can propel you toward your highest good. All you really need to do is listen to what your inner wisdom has to say!

A Course in Miracles

I would like to share the following with you from *A Course in Miracles*. Recite this to yourself every morning, and you will go a long way toward deflecting potential emotional stressors.

Today I make the following commitments:

1. I will not criticize, condemn, complain, or judge.
2. Every decision I make today will be a choice between a grievance and a miracle.
3. I am responsible for what I see, what I choose, and the feelings I experience. I will set goals that I will achieve, and everything that seems to be happening to me I ask for and receive as I have asked.

Getting There

Okay. So now you've learned how to identify different stressors, from environmental to emotional, and you've read about how these stressors can translate into biological afflictions, from malaise to fatal disease. I've also tried to emphasize, again and again, that by reducing these stressors you can create balance in your life. In the big picture, this means simplifying your life, managing time more efficiently, slowing down, nurturing positive attitudes as well as relationships, getting adequate physical activity, and bringing your biological rhythms into balance by following a daily routine. In a much more finite picture, this means using different approaches and treatments, including meditation, yoga, and breathing processes, as well as sensory modulation. Sensory modulation will be covered in chapters to come, but for now let me define it as any therapy that helps create a profound sense of equilibrium and can pacify imbalances in your mindbody physiology. Some examples of these therapies include nutrition, herbal, massage, aroma, color, and sound.

No matter what sorts of stressors are invading your life, know that you can cope with them. You already have the basics, now let's learn how to activate this information.

The Breath of Life

A single wailing breath hails our arrival into this world, just as a single quiet sigh marks our departure. With each inhalation, we take in air molecules that oxygenate our blood and send it coursing through our veins to every cell in our body. When we exhale, we make the grass grow greener, sending carbon dioxide into the environment. It's amazing to think that when we let out a deep breath, we've just exhaled about 10 sextillion air molecules. It takes about six years for one breath to scatter totally throughout the Earth's atmosphere, winding up in faraway places like Paris, Bombay, or Rio de Janeiro. In other words, while you may not be able to afford a glamorous stroll along the Champs Elysée, your breath molecules might be doing just that.

Remembering How to Breathe

In Western industrialized society, few people remember how to breathe correctly. We tend to be shallow chest breathers, and this causes us to subtly hyperventilate, causing our bodily systems and mental processes to

> **Controlling the breath, and thus calming the nerves, is a prerequisite to controlling the mind and the body.**
>
> *Swami Rama*

suffer. On the other hand, when we breathe correctly, this creates an internal rhythm that balances our body organs and systems. How could we become so sloppy about something that should come so naturally? Constant stress causes our muscles to tense and our respiration to increase. Then there's also the issue of "sucking in our gut," a great way to remove perceived inches from your waistline but a definite detriment to your breathing.

The Natural Way

If you observe a sleeping baby, you will witness correct breathing. Watch how the abdomen naturally rises and falls with each breath. A baby makes full use of the diaphragm—that broad muscle sandwiched between the lungs and the abdomen—and not surprisingly, this is called diaphragmatic breathing.

As we live our lives, and unconsciously start to hold life's stresses within the musculoskeletal system, we unconsciously keep the diaphragm frozen. What results are short, shallow breaths.

Return to your beginnings and recapture diaphragmatic breathing. Breathwork, or diaphragmatic breathing, is one of the simplest and most powerful ways to decrease your stress response and increase energy levels in the mindbody physiology. When you bring air down into the lower portion of the lungs, where oxygen exchange is most efficient, your physiology changes dramatically. You receive efficient delivery of oxygen to the brain, muscles, and organs. The heart rate slows down, blood pressure normalizes, digestion improves, tense muscles relax, the busy mind calms down, and unhealthy emotional patterns ease up. In addition, deep breathing can relieve headaches, backaches, stomach aches, and sleeplessness. It helps normalize the body's release of natural painkillers called endorphins. Breathwork has also been shown to help addicts kick the habit—whatever that habit may be. And in one study, diaphragmatic breathing reduced the frequency of hot flashes in menopausal women by 50 percent! Breathing truly is a built-in organic method for healing what ails you.

Check your breathing right now. Put one hand on your chest and one on your abdomen. Inhale and exhale several times. Hopefully one of your hands moved! You actually want your abdomen to extend outward as you bring in a deep, fluid breath. The abdomen then contracts inward as you exhale. This is what diaphragmatic breathing should look like.

Let's Practice Together

You can do diaphragmatic breathing anytime, anywhere. For this exercise, give yourself a quiet space where you'll be undisturbed.

You can stand, sit up straight, or lie down. For the most efficient flow of the life-force energy, you want your spine in alignment.

Bring in a deep breath through your nose. The nose is designed to naturally warm and filter every breath. Feel the flow of this life-giving energy as it travels into and through the length and depth of your lungs. You should feel the lower abdomen moving outward. Visualize every cell in your body receiving this life-giving energy.

As you slowly exhale, your abdomen will move inward. Sense the release of all stress that you may be holding in any part of your body. You should begin to feel a deep sense of relaxation, while at the same time feeling a heightened flow of energy.

Do this exercise at least ten times.

You can heighten the experience by prolonging each inhalation/exhalation, or the length of the overall exercise. Breathwork is an integral part of meditation and visualization, as well as yoga. If you plan to build any of these techniques into your life, be sure to master breathing first.

Moving a step farther, you can also increase your repertoire of breathing capabilities beyond basic diaphragmatic breathing. Breathwork has been explored and documented for centuries—an amazing fact considering that the vast majority of us breathe without thought or consciousness. From all these studies come several important breathing techniques. Let's examine a few of them.

Etch, embroider, or paint the word BREATHE. Frame your artwork and hang it at your workstation. Not only will this serve as a wonderful reminder for you, but I guarantee it will also spur wellness conversations with your clients. It can open the door to a wonderful teaching opportunity as you explain the beauty and health-giving benefits of diaphragmatic breathing. Be sure to explain how breathwork helps control stress and beautify the skin, hair, and nails by providing optimal blood flow through the body. We all can benefit from this information, and we all need gentle reminding. You might want to even add breathing lessons to your salon or spa service menu—no charge, of course!

Pranayama

Diaphragmatic breathing is an integral part of Pranayama. Sanskrit for *science of breath*, this technique focuses on achieving a variety of results for the mindbody physiology, including calming, cooling, and energizing payoffs. There are numerous methods for performing Pranayama, and each has a specific result when seeking balance for the different mind/body constitutions. You may at this point want to refer back to pages 56–60, where we discussed the three energies or mindbody principles of Ayurveda—air, fire, and earth. We'll look at a few Pranayama methods here that may be used for three specific results and benefit anyone.

Got Prana?

Prana is the life-force energy that infuses us when we practice breathwork, creating the calm, alert sense of total integration between mind, body, and spirit. This makes it an excellent breathing foundation for when you practice yoga.

Pranayama: Alternate-Nostril Breathing

This practice is called nadi shodhana. "Nadi" means *channels of circulation*, and "shodhana" means *clearing*. Therefore, this technique helps you clear the channels of circulation, which in turn helps center the mind and relieve tension. Although great for anyone, it is particularly

> Breath is the bridge which connects life to consciousness, which unites your body to your thoughts.
>
> *Thich Naht Hanh*

effective for those with an excess of air energy, quieting an anxious overactive individual. If an overly hectic schedule has you reeling, try nadi shodhana to restore peace of mind. This practice is also calming before meditation.

Sit in a relaxed, comfortable position with a straight spine.

With the mouth closed, use the ring finger of the right hand to close off the left nostril. Inhale smoothly and slowly through the right nostril.

Release the left nostril while closing off the right nostril with the thumb. Exhale slowly and smoothly out of the left nostril.

Now inhale into the left nostril. Breathe diaphragmatically, making the length of each inhalation and exhalation equal.

Close off the left nostril and repeat this cycle of exhalation and inhalation into each nostril several times.

Try to build up to several minutes of this exercise.

Pranayama: Sitali Breath

This practice can be very cooling and soothing for the mindbody physiology, making it an excellent choice for pacifying the fire energy. If you've just had a disagreement with someone and now you're hot under the collar, sitali may help cool you down.

Sit comfortably with the spine straight and eyes closed.

Roll the tongue lengthwise to form a tube. The tip of the tongue will protrude slightly out from the mouth. Inhale smoothly through the rolled tongue, making a hissing sound. Follow the cool sensation down the throat and into the lungs. (If the tongue will not roll lengthwise, roll the tip of the tongue back to touch the soft palate. Inhale through closed teeth, making a hissing sound. Continue with the next step.)

Relaxing the tongue and closing the mouth, exhale fully through the nostrils. Generally the exhale will take slightly longer than the inhale.

Repeat 5 times.

Once proficient with this technique, you may want to extend your practice time.

Pranayama: Kapalabhati Breath

Translated, this means *that which makes the head shine.* This practice is invigorating, so it's a great choice anytime you're feeling lethargic, fatigued, or depressed. It is very effective for balancing the earth energy, as it tends to stimulate the abdominal muscles and digestive organs, massage the internal organs and spinal column, and increase circulation of bodily fluids.

Sit comfortably with the spine straight and eyes closed.

Place the palms of both hands on the abdomen.

Inhale slowly and passively.

Now vigorously and forcefully exhale through the nose, while drawing the stomach tightly inward.

Repeat this passive inhalation and forceful exhalation 10 times.

Once comfortable with the technique, you can use it for up to one minute.

This technique should not be used if you are pregnant or have certain heart conditions.

> **Let** us be silent so that we may hear the whispers of God.
>
> *Ralph Waldo Emerson*

Ujjayi Breath

In Sanskrit, Ujjayi means *control arising from the process of expansion*, and it enhances the ventilation of the lungs, removes congestion, calms the nerves, and energizes the entire body. Yet another part of Pranayama breathwork, this is a practice that helps vitalize the whole body. Because it elicits a certain sound, it is my favorite technique to use when performing yoga, since this sound gently reminds you not to hold your breath while in a posture.

The sound that is made while inhaling and exhaling in Ujjayi is the *ha* sound. To get the hang of this, first try breathing in and out with your mouth open. With the glottis (the opening between the vocal cords in the larynx) at the back of the throat constricted, inhale while making the *ha* sound. Then exhale while making the *ha* sound.

Do you sound like Darth Vader? Then you are doing it right! Whether done for ten breaths, ten minutes, or through a half-hour yoga practice, Ujjayi is a sure-fire way to conjure up free-flowing energy with full awareness.

Meditation

Meditation? Okay, okay, I know some of you think meditation is hocus-pocus. Others of you may already realize the deep power of meditation and its ability to help you perceive the beauty, truth, and goodness in this world. Indeed, I truly believe that meditation is one of the most important practices you can do to manage stress, raise your level of consciousness, and commune with spirit. The results of meditation allow me to more readily witness every action and every thought I have as I'm interacting with my world. With this unbelievable awareness, I have been able to make subtle positive shifts in my thought processes and activities. This practice has brought and continues to bring me such joy. You, too, will experience higher levels of consciousness as you discover the power of meditation. The degree to which this happens, however, is up to you and depends on your level of commitment.

Meditation is one of the most flexible consciousness-raising exercises I've ever come across. It refers to time spent in quiet introspection, and however you can best accomplish this is your form of meditation. You may run, garden, do yoga or tai chi, pray, or perform traditional meditation. As long as a given activity takes you to a place of calm, a place of heightened awareness and energy, a place of heightened clarity of mind, then you are meditating.

In fact, we humans often meditate without even knowing it. Have you ever been absorbed by a beautiful sunset to the exclusion of all other thought? This is a form of meditation. Have you ever been driving along and your mind wanders off, maybe focusing on a problem at home or work? Suddenly you come to a stoplight, and you realize you've driven several miles without even knowing it. This daydreaming is also a form of meditation. Have you ever gotten lost in thought while reading a book, gardening, jogging, working, or even cooking? These are more forms of meditation. Psychologists say that during these lost moments our brain waves are identical to those observed during traditional meditation. While we're in this state, our blood pressure drops, our heart rate goes down, and the immune system receives a powerful boost. Just in from the American Heart Association: meditation apparently serves to strengthen the heart! This finding is based on a study in which individuals meditated for twenty minutes twice a day. After seven months, ultrasounds showed that blockages in their coronary arteries had decreased.

In a society where we tend to ignore internal signals, instead letting external signals rule, it is essential that we give ourselves time to break free and listen to our spirit. Meditation is a practice that can bring us to this place. It can free us from the bondage of our egocentricities and the external influences that prevent us from connecting with our higher selves.

Pure Consciousness

When we transcend our normal waking consciousness and go to a place where we have no thoughts—absolute silence—we experience transcendental or pure consciousness. A very important mentor in my life and an

> **Out beyond ideas of wrongdoing and right doing is a field—I'll meet you there.**
>
> *Rumi*

internationally respected doctor, author, and teacher of mindbody healing, Deepak Chopra, speaks of meditation as going into the *gap*. This is the silent space between thoughts. Please do not think, however, that silence implies lack of action. The *gap* is home to our greatest potentiality and infinite possibilities. This is where we may feel most vividly, most perfectly alive. In this place, you can experience absolute balance and connect with the real you—spirit.

Meditation has been and continues to be an integral part of spiritual traditions worldwide. Somewhat similar to prayer, meditation allows us to feel the intimate presence of a higher power. So how do prayer and meditation differ? Deepak explains this beautifully: "When you are praying, you are speaking to God, when in meditation, you are listening to God." I find this statement to be quite profound, and it puts many things into perspective for me. Both activities are important and at the heart of our spirituality, allowing us to feel the intimate presence of a higher power.

Meditation has changed my perception of things. I find myself more flexible and accepting. Along with my daily breathing practices, it is how I reduce stress and find inner peace. You must want to have these benefits in your life before you can realize a true commitment to meditation. Just as with physical exercise, there should be no compromise on meditation time. Make it as important and integral to your day as bathing, eating, and sleeping. Coming to meditation from this perspective, you will experience great richness.

Mantra

A mantra is a particular sound that you use to reach your place of silence. My mantra was chosen according to the vibrational sound of the universe at the time and place of my birth. It was determined by Vedic mathematics (the Vedas are the four ancient, sacred texts of Hinduism). You may also choose as your mantra any word or sound that has personal meaning. The unique vibrational quality of a mantra allows you to fluidly take your awareness into a deep inner silence where pure consciousness resides. When this happens, mental activity decreases along with overall biochemical activity. This gives the body a profound rest.

While I highly recommend setting a regular time every day for meditation, you may also want to meditate for shorter periods of time during different parts of the day. These brief meditations provide moments to regroup when stress reaches hysterical peaks or energy hits unbearable lows. You probably will not go to your deepest, most peaceful place, but nonetheless, these can be extremely helpful times. Consider a brief two-minute breathing exercise, a walk in nature, a private moment to daydream out the office window, a few minutes spent in a serenity garden, or simply five silent minutes between clients. All are valid and viable ways to bring the benefits of meditation into your life. You will all find your own way to meditation. To get started, try listing five methods and practices that might prove conducive to quiet time.

_____

_____

_____

_____

_____

_____

_____

Now think back over your day and write down five times when a brief meditative moment might have provided a quick respite and a healthier response to life.

_____

_____

_____

_____

_____

_____

_____

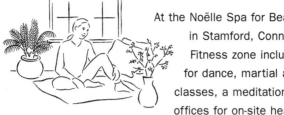 At the Noëlle Spa for Beauty and Wellness in Stamford, Connecticut, a Spiritual Fitness zone includes studio space for dance, martial arts, and yoga classes, a meditation room, and offices for on-site health practitioners. These practitioners include a naturopath, a gynecologist, and a registered dietitian and nutritionist.

At the Chopra Center for Well Being in La Jolla, California, health is seen as higher consciousness, and thus there is an on-site meditation room. Here guests and staff alike go for reflection between Ayurvedic beauty and wellness therapies, medical consultations, satsangs, and visits to the organic café.

These are two shining examples of how beauty and wellness companies successfully integrate wellness services and products with more traditional beauty services.

Is there a space in your salon or spa that could be designated as a meditation room? Where is it? What changes would you need to make to this location?

_____

_____

_____

_____

_____

_____

_____

_____

_____

_____

_____

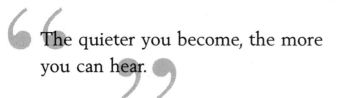

The quieter you become, the more you can hear.

Ram Dass

Meditation in Practice

Ideally, you should give yourself the gift of meditation at least twice a day, 20 minutes per session. Consider meditating at dawn and dusk, when the vibration of our circadian rhythms are most calm and peaceful. Sunrise meditation allows you to carry a sense of clarity and calmness into your workday. Sunset meditation brings you to your sleeping consciousness prepared for potentially vivid and inspiring dreams.

Choose a place that is quiet and comfortable. You will want to feel protected when meditating. If you create a tranquil atmosphere, the mind will soften and focus more readily. Make this a special place with comfortable cushions to support your lower back and knees (necessary if sitting in the easy sitting posture, legs crossed), natural, organic, scented candles (no lead wicks, please), incense or essential oils, and a personal altar if desired. Do anything you like to enhance the sacred atmosphere where you go to connect with spirit.

Make yourself feel comfortable. If it feels right, wrap yourself in a shawl or blanket during meditation. This can create a feeling of protection and reduce any sensations of vulnerability.

You may use a personal mantra, as we discussed, a chant, or simply become aware of your breath.

To calm and center yourself before beginning meditation, consider doing a few minutes of alternate-nostril breathing or diaphragmatic breathing, alone or coupled with yoga postures.

Sit in a chair with your spine in a natural and straight position, sit on the floor in a lotus position, or sit in a cross-legged position. If you need back support, sit on a rolled towel or cushion. Ultimately you want to strengthen the back, abdominal, pelvic, and leg muscles so you can sit through meditation for any length of time without discomfort. Many yoga books, videos, and classes specifically address this issue. One of my favorites is *Yoga: Mastering the Basics* (Himalayan Institute Press).

Now close your eyes and bring your attention to your breathing. Breathe deeply, smoothly, and naturally. Pay attention to the in-flow and out-flow of your breath. Do not try to alter or control the breath. If you are distracted by thoughts floating through your mind, sounds in the

> *In a pure mind there is constant awareness of the Self; freedom ends bondage and joy ends sorrow.*
>
> *Chandogya Upanishad*

surrounding environment, or sensations in the body, that's all right. Let them come and go as you bring your attention back to the breath.

Continue this process for anywhere up to 20 minutes. At the end of this time, slowly and gently open your eyes. Bring your awareness back to your surroundings.

Am I Doing This Right?

What you just read is an outline of one traditional way to meditate. Please understand that you may meditate wherever you are, at any time, and in any way you choose. Really, the only time I do not recommend meditation is when you are driving a vehicle.

No matter where, when, why, or how you meditate, you should know that there is no wrong way to do it. If you find yourself falling asleep, it's okay. It indicates that you are tired! If you find yourself fending off a barrage of thoughts, it's okay. It indicates that you have a lot on your mind and probably need to release these thoughts before they turn into harmful stress. Let the thoughts come and go. As for finding the right way to access the silence we discussed, trust me! You will find it. All you need to do is show up with the intention and you will experience an awakening to the miracle of existence.

Making the Connection

Consider any and all of these consciousness-raising practices discussed in this chapter to reduce stress and increase your ability to connect with spirit.

Become as mindful as possible, witnessing everything that you do. Observe yourself reading this sentence right now. When you shower, really feel the water on your skin. When you eat, really taste your food. When you perform a beauty service, really be with the client and every nuance of the service being performed. When you crawl into bed tonight, observe yourself shifting from wakefulness to sleep.

Commit to the power of breathing exercises, meditation, positive affirmations, creative visualization, and physical activities such as yoga, tai chi,

> The external harmony and progress of the entire human race is founded on the internal harmony and progress of every individual.
>
> *Maharishi Mahesh Yogi*

pilates, or dance. Each practice serves to hone our sensitivity and mindfulness, allowing our spirit to soar into uncharted waters—into the realm of infinite possibilities.

Get lost in organic and sacred rituals. Burn a favorite candle or incense, then connect with the scent and color and movement of the flame. Play enchanting music, then hear each individual note as well as the harmony. Read your favorite poetry aloud and listen to the rhyme and texture of the words.

Walk in nature. Enjoy the sensual feast inherent in everything. See the smallest details in the leaves, rocks, and water. See the universe in a leaf. Feel the sun on your face, and the wind in your hair. Listen to nature's primordial sounds. Look for the man in the moon.

Create a thing of beauty. As beauty professionals we exert great thought and care toward making our clients feel beautiful. Expand your creativity into other realms. Sketch, paint, mold clay, make a mosaic or ornament. Get lost in the process. Whatever it is that you create exemplifies organic beauty.

Construct an altar at home or work. Whether on a windowsill or upon a huge oak table, place things here that have special meaning for you—a loved one's photo, a lock of hair, a feather, a rosary, or perhaps a quartz gem. Every time you see this altar, you are gently reminded of spirit's presence, and you should feel calmer and more centered.

Let your soul write. Keep a journal each and every day. Write down whatever is on your mind, without editing or censoring. You will experience so many insights.

Cultivate peace in a garden. This can involve an acre out back or a terra-cotta pot on your veranda. Visualize what your garden will look like after it receives loving care, then set out to bring this beauty home. See your garden as a metaphor for your inner garden: planting, weeding, and harvesting.

Know that you are beauty personified. Spend a day on yourself, indulging in beautifying rituals. Visit a spa. Let a cadre of other beauty professionals nurture you and treat you to an experience of sheer bliss. Along similar lines, you might invite a friend over and perform beautifying rituals on each other.

Tune in to the cosmic rhythms of the universe—the calendar of the soul. Honor the sun, the moon, and the stars. Celebrate the seasons. Is it spring, with blossoms bursting open and a general resurgence of energy everywhere? See this as a metaphor for your mindbody physiology. Is it winter, when life returns into the soil for a season of deep introspection? Another great metaphor to feed into.

Honor every significant stage in your life, as well as momentous stages in your loved ones' lives. This may mean something as seemingly small as cutting out one hour of television every night so you can find quiet time to meditate, as well as huge events like giving birth, getting married, or losing a loved one. Honor them all!

We've covered a lot of ground so far, with a lot of ideas and practices that will help you become more aware of the life-force energy that surrounds and permeates all of creation. These are all ways to create balance. How are you faring so far? I sincerely hope you're enjoying the ride.

Notes:

Chapter Five

Mindfulness in Motion

Few seem conscious that there is
such a thing as physical morality.

Hippocrates

This chapter, as part of our journey toward career consciousness, delves into the realm of movement. Let me say right up front that the purpose of this chapter is *not* to teach you exercises. There are already magnificently illustrated books out there, as well as plenty of reputable personal fitness consultants, yoga teachers, and movement therapists to help you work with your body and its specific needs. This chapter is about the true nature of physical movement, beginning with various categories of physical movement that can serve to enhance our personal lives and careers. Then we'll move on to a better appreciation of conscious movement, or how ergonomically correct body movements, especially when coupled with stretching exercises, can serve to maximize productivity by minimizing body fatigue and discomfort. Being mindful of your movements means so much to us as beauty and wellness professionals. By chapter's end, I think you'll see how a combination of physical activity and conscious movement leads us ever closer to our quest for harmony between the multidimensional layers of self—body, mind, and spirit.

Making the Connection

Now for a bit of philosophical stuff. Pay close attention, my friends.

Movement is what connects intention to action. When we are sedentary, our intentions become disconnected from our actions. It is then, in this state of physical inactivity, that we risk losing one of our most precious gifts—spontaneity. This loss makes it difficult to engage joyfully and passionately in any effort toward fulfillment of our goals.

Moreover, a chasm, or disconnect, between thought and action may result in inertia and profound fatigue. It sounds illogical that nonmovement could create fatigue, but it is a fact. Exercise, the regular, deliberate, and pleasurable physical movement of the body, can help stave off this inertia. We'll talk in a bit about the biochemistry of exercise and its wholly admirable qualities.

If we forsake regular physical movement and disconnect our intentions from our actions, depression or at least some aspects of this debilitating mental illness become a real possibility. It's like that old saying: the mind is willing but the body is not. When this happens, we tend to give up, making ourselves prime targets for despondency, melancholy . . . depression!

What's more, without spontaneity and conscious movement, daily tensions may gain the upper hand, lacing the body and psyche in a sort of straitjacket. Fascia, the connective tissue that surrounds and encases our muscles, can form harmful holding patterns. Think about the hurts, strains, sprains, and pains we experience when we become passive about our activity or our life force. Simply standing up from the couch can be a strain for the couch potato. Merely walking across the room for anyone who is physically inactive could produce an ankle blowout. So many people currently wear this metaphoric straightjacket that antidotes have been developed for it. One type of remedy is Myofacial Release, a form of bodywork created specifically to disengage these fixed patterns in one's fascia. Rolfing is another well-known approach.

If left unattended, stress, physical or mental, begins to prevent free-flowing movement into new thought processes and positions. The mind starts to establish parameters beyond which we are not allowed to move. Only certain movements and only certain habits are permitted. Over time, we can suffer debilitating diseases—physically and emotionally. Regular free-flowing and spontaneous movement can and will release you from this type of stranglehold. Have I gotten your full attention yet? Good! I realize this is intense, but it is also real. So for goodness sake, get moving!

> **The** sovereign invigorator of the
> body is exercise.

Thomas Jefferson

Here's another piece of real news, and it's all good. Pleasurable, glorious exercise is a primary way to ignite, renew, or maintain the vital link between our intentions and our actions . . . our spontaneous and joyful love of life.

Our Physicality

Of course, when I say that we all need to get physical, I am not recommending that we all become triathletes. As a beauty professional, you instinctively know what's good for you and what your physicality can endure. You know because you're tested daily! Maybe for you this endurance test means cutting 10 to 15 heads of hair a day, giving 5 to 6 full-body massages, or 8 to 12 facials, providing 12 to 15 manicures, making countless phone calls, spending too many hours on the computer, or meeting, greeting, and treating a myriad of clients. Perhaps we should consider ourselves beauty athletes!

Following this train of thought, I can't stress enough how important fitness is when it comes to not only making it through all these challenges, but making it through with joy. Striving toward your own physical fitness, along with conscious movements throughout the day, will help you win the race, deflecting stress, and staving off fatigue and injuries while sustaining high energy levels. When you accomplish all this, you leave yourself wide open to experience your wholeness and thus your beauty.

Fortunately, the magnificent bodies that our spirits reside in are designed to find balance between motion and stillness, exercise and relaxation. But we do need to be conscious—to really know our body—in order for the body to do its job.

The Real Deal

Every moment that you devote to consistent and regular physical activity is a blessing for the body, mind, and soul. Our well-being depends on physical activity. It is, along with proper nutrition, one of the greatest healers. It is also one of the best beautifiers. Think about how beautiful

> **The human body has one ability not possessed by any machine—the ability to repair itself.**
>
> *George E. Kirley Jr., M.D.*

you look after any physical activity. After completing a brief lunchtime walk, look in the mirror. I bet you'll see that an inviting smile has replaced that mid-morning harried scowl. How beautiful is that! And how about your skin's natural luminescence after a more strenuous 30-minute workout? No amount of blush can produce such a radiant glow!

Your body, as an expression of spirit, is most blissful when moving with the life force flowing through it, whether working, dancing, stretching, performing or any form of natural movement, for that matter.

Did Your "Get Up and Go" Get Up and Leave?

According to the Surgeon General, only 26 percent of the U.S. population exercises regularly. This is woeful! In a society so sedentary, none of these facts is surprising:

- Many of us feel spiritually deprived.
- Depression is more prevalent than ever, with an estimated 19 million Americans suffering some form of depression.
- One-third of the American population is obese, or at least 20 percent over their acceptable weight. This remains true despite the fat figure of 40 billion dollars a year being poured into anything and everything connected to weight loss.
- The rise in childhood obesity is tracking upward at an alarming pace.

Are all these facts manifestations of a crisis in consciousness? Why is it that so many of us forfeit health and happiness and instead choose a love affair with the couch and TV? How could such a

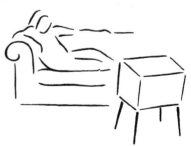

> "Health is the vital principle of bliss,
> and exercise, of health.
>
> *James Thomson*

collectively intelligent population as ours become so fat and out of shape? Why, this epidemic even has a name—sedentary death syndrome. Yes, it's true! Frank W. Booth, a professor at the University of Missouri-Columbia, coined the term in order to lend this chronic and potentially fatal condition credibility, and thus hopefully to make the federal government pay more attention and devote more funding to getting America back on its feet.

A recent medical study conducted at Columbia Children's Hospital in Ohio confirmed that today's children are heavier and have significantly higher cholesterol and triglyceride levels than kids did fifteen years ago. One of the researchers, Dr. Hugh Allens, said, "Unless these trends change, 30 million of the 80 million children alive today in the United States will eventually die of heart disease . . . Kids need to turn off the TV, get off the couch, and stop the nincompooping of America."

When you are with your children, try to set a good example. You are their role model. Know that your attitudes and actions most definitively play a role in the habits your children may form. For working parents, this is sometimes easier said than done, since you are not always in your children's presence, but you can resolve to be in the moment when at work, and then certainly be in the moment when at home with your loved ones. When you are with the kids, replace high-fat junk food with good nutritional stuff. Turn off the TV, computer, or CD player and get the kids exercising. Walk, bike, play catch, hike, whatever floats your boat—and do it consistently. Oh, yes. Don't forget to join them. You're the pacesetter for your children's healthy life.

Five Easy Pieces

Mark Twain once said, "Oh, I get the urge to exercise every now and then, but I just lay down 'til it goes away." Now, you may find this amusing, as did I, but in reality, I know you will find physical exercise far *more*

> You have to stay in shape. My grandmother, she started walking five miles a day when she was 60. She's 97 today and we don't know where the hell she is.
>
> *Ellen DeGeneres*

entertaining. Or should I say, you will enjoy the way physical activity helps balance the mindbody physiology. It feels so good; it feels so right; it is what our bodies are meant to do.

To help you discover this joy, I offer five easy steps.

1. Your first step toward discovering the true amusement of physical activity is to change your mind-set. Too many of us view exercise as drudgery, something to get through as quickly as possible, a punishment. Instead, see it as a delectable dessert. Yes, I know many of you are already coming from this place, but a much larger percentage of you are not. If you are not exercising adequately or often enough for your mindbody physiology's needs (and desires), it will come back to haunt you through all sorts of maladies. Okay, okay, I'll get off my rant here. But I'm not making this stuff up.

2. The second step so many of us need to take before we can truly learn to enjoy physical activity is finding time. Time always seems to be a primary reason for not exercising. If you can begin to see how physical activity can dramatically change your mindbody physiology, it will become a priority. You may even be amazed at how many minutes you find for a little stretching here and a little walking there. And a bit here and there does count. Ten morning minutes on your treadmill, a brisk walk after lunch, a few yoga stretches between clients, a little more yoga when you get home at night . . . it all does cumulative good, and it all counts.

And if you don't like structured physical activity, be creative. Dance free-form in your living room. Wash the kitchen floor to a beat. If your passion is shopping, make yourself walk the entire mall before buying that yummy suede jacket. Exercise is as important as good nutrition, restful sleep, brushing and flossing your teeth, healthy sex . . . Whoops, there goes that rant again! But I really want

> Here in this body are the sacred rivers: here are the sun and the moon, as well as all the pilgrimage places. I have not encountered another temple as blissful as my own body.
>
> *Saraha*

you to understand that the feel-good benefits of consistent structured or free-flowing exercise are huge.

3. I think I've made my point about how good exercise is for us. Not to worry, no rant coming on! Instead, I want to gently steer you back to a few vital tools we already discussed, specifically certain techniques that can actualize introspection and attitudinal changes. Applying these techniques to your attitude about exercise is the third step in learning to appreciate physical activity.

Try using your visualization skills to image yourself through the stages of life that lie before you. Perhaps you can visualize yourself during the golden years—75, or 80, 85 or 90—still taking that early-morning swim, pedaling to the marketplace, or briskly walking a few miles each morning. See how healthy, vigorous, and energetic you feel, enjoying every moment of every day. Contrast this with an image of yourself as an overweight, bedridden, and constantly fatigued elder who truly feels old. No, you say? You can't or won't imagine this miserable scenario? Okay, this is the first step in making your move. Stick with the beautiful, healthy visual. It just might inspire you to begin or maintain your dedication to a daily regimen of physical activity.

4. Reading this page marks your fourth step toward learning to love physical activity—because once you finish the following paragraph, you will have knowledge. You will understand how regular exercise literally benefits every physical and mental process. On a sweeping level, it enhances our energy and stamina levels—a biggie for us beauty pros. It also enhances the immune system, which is, again, so important for the beauty professional. Think about how many people you meet, how many bodies you touch, and how many of these people are just getting over or just coming down with a cold.

Moving on to specifics, physical activity benefits your heart and your blood vessels, your musculoskeletal system, and your respiration. It is key in managing or reducing weight. Your entire body benefits from regular movement. These benefits include improved cardiovascular and respiratory function, which results in the enhanced transport of oxygen and nutrients to every cell in the body. Activity also enhances the movement of carbon dioxide and waste products from the tissues of the body into the bloodstream and on to the eliminative organs—whether through perspiration, urination, or bowel movements. Metabolic wastes and lactic acid collect in our bodies when we stop moving. This further supports the claim that regular exercise can be one of the most powerful rituals for detoxification.

As discussed elsewhere, we need to protect and support all our body's natural and constant detoxification systems, so as not to accumulate toxins in our mindbody physiology. How comforting to know that we can enhance the detox process through consistent physical activity.

5. Had a bad day? Here's your fifth and final reason to love exercise! Physical activity has the power to improve your mood and your ability to handle or relieve stress. It constructively counters cortisol and other fight-or-flight hormones that are released during high-stress situations. In addition, those who exercise regularly have been shown to have higher self-esteem and a generally happier outlook. Perhaps you've heard of the runner's high? This occurs because exercise triggers a release of endorphins, which induce tremendous exhilaration. The resulting elevation of mood may last for anywhere from 90 to 120 minutes after completing an exercise session. The increase in our basal metabolic rate hums on well past that.

From your mood to your metabolism, your heart to your immune system, your muscles to your bones . . . it's just the cat's meow, so delicious and delectable is exercise.

P.S. There are loads of additional reasons I love physical activity, but these are more personal—it gets me out of the house, I meet great people, it gives me something interesting to talk about, it helps me sleep, it enhances my sex life. . . . Look for reasons unique to you and treasure them!

> *If we all did the things we are capable of doing, we would literally astound ourselves.*
>
> *Thomas Edison*

Use this page as an exercise journal. Answer the following questions, add your own spontaneous thoughts, then go take a walk!

What are your exercise habits? Describe them in terms of intensity, frequency, and duration.

_____

_____

_____

_____

How often do you put in a little extra physical activity time and what forms does it take? For example, do you take the stairs instead of the elevator? Do you ever park in the farthest space or down a side street and then walk to the salon entrance? Do you go by foot instead of car when doing neighborhood errands?

_____

_____

_____

_____

What physical activities do you enjoy most?

_____

_____

_____

_____

Where are some lovely places you might enjoy walking, biking, jogging, or rollerblading?

_____

_____

_____

_____

What inspires you to get up and get going?

_____

_____

_____

_____

What incentives or rewards might help you maintain a regular exercise regime? (Make these incentives realistic, and if you do get up and go, don't forget to give yourself the promised reward!)

_____

_____

_____

_____

Do you have any pals who might enjoy brisk buddy-walks with you?

_____

_____

_____

_____

List other ideas to get yourself motivated.

_____

_____

_____

_____

Optimal Movement

For those of you who get physical at your training heart rate for at least 20 minutes three times a week, congratulations! You are receiving cardiovascular benefits from exercise. Ideally, though, it is best to make exercise a part of your daily routine in whatever way you possibly can. A new study published in the *Journal of the American Medical Association* suggests that sedentary people who perform a total of 30 minutes of moderate-intensity physical activity most days of the week will experience significant physical changes (i.e., lower blood pressure and blood cholesterol levels and a healthier body composition). If you have been sedentary, confer with your doctor before beginning a regular program.

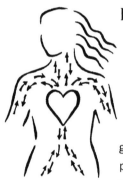

Love Thy Heart

We spoke of the heart in a previous chapter, discussing how your heart is the seat of human emotion, especially as it relates to compassion and loving-kindness. Now I urge you to give some of this compassion and loving-kindness back to your heart. Regularly get physical. In an average life span, the heart pumps blood around our body 2,755,720,800 times. Through exercise, we strengthen this amazing muscle and the vascular system through which all your blood flows. Studies show that an unfit person has a risk of heart attack or stroke that is eight times greater than that of someone who is physically fit. As for the outer dimension of our beauty, the more efficiently our nutrient-rich blood circulates, the more beautiful and healthy our skin, hair, nails, and eyes will be.

Types of Physical Activity

There are three types of physical activity that we may indulge in: aerobic activity for cardiovascular fitness, stretching for flexibility, and weight-bearing activities for strengthening. Every possible physical activity falls within one of these three categories or combines them. Ideally, you want your physical activities to strike a balance between all three.

Aerobic activity enhances cardiovascular fitness. It reduces blood pressure and the possibility of coronary heart disease, decreases the resting heart rate and increases aerobic work capacity, and thus endurance. It can also decrease body fat, increase HDL (the "good cholesterol") bolster the immune system, and, overall, improve your quality of life. In addition, cardiovascular fitness can greatly reduce stress. For every one hour of aerobic activity, there is reportedly a two-hour increase in longevity. Consider brisk walking, jogging, swimming, biking, skiing, dancing, and power yoga.

Flexibility exercises, or stretching movements, allow for greater freedom of movement and improved posture. Stretching will also increase physical and mental relaxation and is great for releasing muscle tension and soreness. It is recommended that stretching be done before (warm-up) and after (cool-down) any form of cardio workout. This reduces injury risks. Stretching is also important if you sit or stand for lengthy periods. Take a delicious stretch whenever you have a free moment and look into activities that enhance flexibility, including yoga, tai chi, and Pilates. These forms of movement are very effective in helping us connect the mind, body, and spirit. Concentrating on your breath while moving through these types of activities brings us face to face with our intrinsic source of energy.

Strengthening or weight-bearing activities are integral to a balanced fitness program. They enhance your power, endurance, and coordination. Strength training will build muscle tone and mass. Muscle tissue is partly responsible for the number of calories burned at rest (the basal metabolic rate, or BMR). As muscle mass increases, BMR increases, making it easier to maintain a healthy body weight. So along with the aesthetic benefits of looking lean and toned, this type of exercise allows your body to burn fat more efficiently. In addition, it strengthens muscles and connective tissue and may ward off osteoporosis. As your strength increases, it will require less effort to perform daily activities—at home or work. You may choose to use free weights, weight machines, or elastic bands. You may also participate in weight-bearing activities such as brisk walking and yoga.

Meditation in Motion

The more you relax while working out, the more efficiently you build muscle and burn fat. When tense, you tighten muscles that should stay slack, your movements become wooden, and you tire faster. Breath awareness and use of a mantra are both simple ways to help you relax and bring full awareness into your physical activity. Silently repeat a favorite word, use Ujjayi breath (see page 86), and focus intently on your movements. Your workout will benefit tremendously from these extra measures.

Consider these ways to enhance your mindfulness in motion:

- *Walking*—Lean forward, just a touch, from the ankles. This helps you pick up speed. Be careful, however, not to lean forward from the waist! Swing your arms with power. This helps propel the opposite leg forward, gives your upper body a better workout, and helps you gain speed.

- *Running*—Smile. Grimacing can make you clench your jaw, which in turn tightens your muscles and hampers your breathing. As you smile, drop your shoulders and roll your head around to dissolve tightness.

- *Bicycling*—Pedal fast, about 80 to 90 revolutions a minute, to burn the most calories. Practice by shifting into an easy gear and pedaling to the count of one potato, two potato, three potato. Work on pedaling smoothly.

- *Weight-lifting*—Get the most out of a set by keeping your movements fluid. Breathe deeply. Don't jerk, and don't rest at the halfway point. If you're bench pressing, lift evenly all the way to the top and, without hesitating, bring the weights slowly back down to your chest.

- *Swimming*—Refine your technique and you'll go farther faster. The best arm stroke is one that follows an S-shape: swing your arm wide as it moves past your shoulder, then bring it back in under your chest, and finally back out again past your hip.

Exercise, Ayurvedically Speaking

Exercise is a major element of a daily Ayurvedic balancing routine, serving to balance your mindbody constitution or type.

The air constitution benefits greatly from calming low-impact activities that focus on agility and coordination. Stretching, yoga, swimming, brisk walking, light bicycling, and gentle dancing are a few possibilities.

Fire constitutions, who tend to be competitive by nature, should avoid competitive sports and lean instead toward moderate activity. Yoga, swimming, jogging, bicycling, hiking, weight-lifting, tennis, racquetball, and skiing are a few suggestions.

Earth constitutions, with bodies built for endurance, do well with more intense exercise such as power yoga, jogging, strenuous weight training, swimming, vigorous bicycling or spinning, aerobic dance of any kind, cross-country skiing, and basically any aerobic activity.

Become a Physical Activist

The key to developing a regular regimen of physical activity is finding the optimal intensity, frequency, and duration of exercise for you. Intensity is how hard you exercise, taking into consideration the pace at which you run or walk and the amount of weight you lift, as well as your heart rate when involved in any form of organized exercise. Frequency is how often you exercise, taking into consideration how many days or sessions you exercise per week. Duration is how many minutes you perform an activity; it can also mean the number of sets, or repetitions, you perform in weight training. Your body will let you know if you're overreaching in any of these areas. Warm up, cool down, don't go beyond where your body wants you to go, and your body will cooperate.

If you're not sure about what's right for your particular body, there are highly qualified fitness professionals to consult. Look for these experts at local health clubs, a community college, or through fitness centers aligned with your hospital. You definitely want a degreed or certified fitness professional. Certification should come from IDEA (International Association of Fitness Professionals), the leading organization serving personal trainers, exercise instructors, and business operators. Check out their excellent website www.ideafit.com. Another reputable certification might come from ACE (American Council on Exercise).

When you do find the right personal fitness professional, be prepared to answer lots of questions pertaining to your daily routine and what you hope to accomplish. Also, be ready to discuss your regular eating habits (honestly!), since your fitness expert will most likely want to know about your nutritional level. Don't forget to ask about classes. The fitness center at my community hospital offers try-me classes, a great idea if you are not yet sure which type of physical activity—cardiovascular, flexibility, or strengthening—is best suited for your mindbody physiology.

There are also excellent videos and books that may supply a few answers, but personal one-on-one attention is probably best.

Last but certainly not least, if you have been sedentary for a long time, I definitely recommend conferring with your primary care physician prior to beginning any regular fitness program.

You, as well as the salon or spa where you work, may want to consider setting up a referral system with your community fitness center and local personal fitness trainers. Bring one or a few of these experts into your salon or spa for an all-staff informational session. Ask your experts to discuss personal fitness as well as fitness on the job.

Consider arranging an evening session, and if the space allows, have the staff go through a fitness routine with your fitness professional. Perhaps key into movements that can easily be done during breaks and in between clients. Look at the simple stretches at the end of this chapter, and use them!

Don't forget to share your referral list with clients, too! Who isn't looking for a highly recommended exercise class!?! In addition to referrals, you might consider hosting a fitness-geared event for clients. This could include actual activities or consist strictly of an informational session.

You Gotta Love Yoga

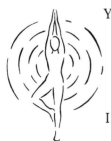
You may have noticed that yoga showed up in all three physical activity types. The intensity or gentleness of your yoga practice, along with the speed with which you perform each yoga move, determines the overall benefits of a yoga session. Regardless of which yoga style you choose, I think you'll enjoy it. I know I do! I *love* my yoga.

Yoga works on a deep and profound level, and while some of you may already understand the magic I refer to, others might need a brief introduction. Thus, I want to devote a little special time to this extraordinary practice.

Whether or not you live it, you probably at least know of yoga. It's become quite popular here in the U.S. We Americans, however, tend to physicalize yoga, working through asanas, or postures. We tend to regard it primarily in terms of its fitness component. This is valid; it is one of my primary physical activities, coupled with regular brisk walks. But yoga can go much farther, becoming a lifestyle. (We'll discuss this in a moment.) In addition, there are many types of yoga to discover—Hatha, Integral, Sivananda, Ashtanga, Bikram, Iyengar, and Kundalini, to name but a few. Also, there are thousands of yoga postures to luxuriate in. To make a long story short, when it comes to yoga philosophy and asanas, you could go a lifetime and never run out of things to learn!

I'll do my best in the next few pages to provide a quick journey through the history, virtues, and possibilities of yoga.

A Philosophy to Live By

To begin at the beginning, yoga has been around for over 5,000 years. An ancient Hindu practice, literally meaning "union" or "yoke," it represents a philosophy for living one's life. In Ayurveda, it is seen as a concept intertwining the mind, body, and spirit in a mutually supportive relationship. This holistic lifestyle weaves together fitness, wellness, and consciousness-raising. It nurtures the flow of the life-force energy, or prana, throughout our mindbody physiology.

What does all this weaving, intertwining, and connectivity accomplish? A lot! Western studies show that those who practice yoga regularly are less anxious and more resistant to stress. These people tend to have lower blood pressure and more efficient heart function. One research study suggests that yoga can cut asthma attacks by up to 75 percent, and reduce the amount of insulin needed by diabetics. Studies at the National Institutes of Health found a strong correlation between yoga and the clearing of the coronary arteries, as well as some proof that yoga postures and breathing techniques can significantly control back injuries, along with arthritis and rheumatism.

In addition to benefiting the body, yoga also greatly benefits the mind—of course, this makes perfect sense, since the mind and body are really one. Some call their yoga practice "meditation in motion," and it can indeed have a meditative effect by virtue of the concentration you place on your breath while performing postures. Its simultaneous ability to calm and invigorate results in a distinct heightening of your awareness.

As yoga serves to increase the body's flexibility, promote better blood circulation (with all the significant benefits that accompany this), speed up metabolism, and improve digestion, as well as enhance endocrine and organ functions, it helps us to fully realize our inner and outer beauty. Our minds calm down, our limbs become long and lean, and our mindbody physiology functions from a place of wholeness. We radiate this vibrant energy.

Yoga is also a most flexible physical activity—pun intended! It's a wonderful activity to perform on its own or as an adjunct to other activities. Alone, it can provide a complete workout, balancing and aligning every part of you, including muscles, bones, and breath. Depending on the speed and length at which you perform yoga, it can be a cardio workout, as in Ashtanga or Bikram yoga. Also, like weight lifting, yoga can strengthen the muscles through resistance exercises, except instead of using barbells and machines, you use your body's own weight. Isometric exercises, like weight lifting and yoga, are useful for the same purpose.

Optimally, yoga is combined with Pranayama, or breathing techniques. And it is ideal for preparing to go into meditation, quieting the mind and bringing awareness inward into the silence—where you commune with spirit.

As for the best time of day to practice yoga, any time is the right time. Personally, I enjoy practicing yoga in the early morning before getting out of bed—yes, bed yoga! I also practice a flow of postures, requiring about 20 to 30 minutes, before I hit the treadmill, cross-country ski machine, or the great outdoors. I've also been known to practice it in the evening, especially when my work takes me traveling. Alone at night in a hotel room, yoga is a wonderful way to unwind and maybe shake off a little homesickness for my husband and pooches.

Please know that you don't have to do a lengthy yoga practice each and every day to realize the benefits. To optimize yoga's delicious powers of mindbody rejuvenation, daily practice is most important, and one, two, or three postures at a time can do the trick. Whether in the salon between clients, at home before you take a walk, or as a cardio workout warm-up, a few postures will provide tremendous benefit. Consistent use of a few basic postures goes a long way toward loosening up physical constraints and opening yourself up to new possibilities of mental and emotional experience. A condensed routine could include a forward bend, a backward bend, and a twist.

Yoga-tizing the Workday

If you can, steal a few moments between clients to do the grounding ritual we talked about earlier coupled with a yoga posture or two— maybe yoga for the wrists, a forward bend, an inversion (modified shoulder stand), or the child's pose. You can do many of these seated in a chair, or if room exists, certainly perform them fully on the floor. I'm all for every salon or spa having a yoga or meditation space. In fact, there are some amazing state-of-the-art spas and salons that include yoga studios in their environment.

If you wish to integrate a mindbody fitness area into your salon or spa but you're short on space, consider checking out some of the new salon furniture options that can be wheeled around. By wheeling salon stations and chairs out of the way, you can clear a space for staff members to sit comfortably on the floor and perform yoga. Believe me, your mobile furniture investment will come back to reward you with healthier, happier, more productive employees.

The Asanas or Postures

As mentioned, there are thousands of postures, or asanas. These postures fall into six basic types: standing postures, inversions, backbends, forward bends, twists, and meditational postures. This last group is used in between more difficult postures, and definitely at the end of a yoga session. You do not want to leap up right after your yoga practice and dash back into activity. You want to lie in a meditational posture for at least five minutes—allowing your mind and body time to fully experience the enhanced energy flow and the heightened consciousness that have just been generated through your practice.

Breathe!

As in all exercise, a key to yoga is remembering to breathe—smoothly and evenly. Called Pranayama, our vital energy flows freely through breath. As a guideline, you want to inhale when extending the body and exhale when flexing the body. And certainly when holding a posture for any length of time, breathe smoothly, fluidly, and diaphragmatically.

Stay True to Yourself

The golden rule for all yoga enthusiasts, especially those of us attending classes, is to never, ever be competitive. If you find yourself trying to match or one-up your teacher or the person on the mat beside you, then you've unfortunately missed the point. Move to your own rhythm . . . to your own physical limits. Concentrate only on your own body and breathwork. This deep focus allows your body to fully let go and sink deeper into a posture. And, yes, this can be the most delicious release!

Plenty of Resources

Speaking of classes, I encourage you to take one. Or look into the many excellent audiotapes, videos, and television shows that are offered. *Lilias!*, hosted by Lilias Folan, is one of my favorite television shows, and can be seen on many PBS stations. She's been on TV doing yoga since I was a kid (which was many moons ago), and here she is today, as beautiful, serene, and limber as ever. Living Arts is exceptional in the quality of their educational videos. *Yoga Journal* and *Yoga International* are excellent monthly magazines that keep you abreast of current developments in the realm of yoga. I also suggest you check out www.yogasite.com, a great website for information, links, and articles. So many excellent resources exist—I've listed some of my favorites in the resource section.

Everybody Dance

Mindful or serenity-generating exercise programs (yoga among them) are very popular right now. The aging Baby Boomer population, coupled with the world's spiritual awakening, has greatly impacted this trend. Yoga, tai

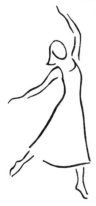

chi, Pilates, and the many other stretch/relaxation workouts out there—they are all about slowing down and finding balance. They are what you could call total-awareness workouts or stress-free fitness activities.

One particular kind of total-awareness workout is dance. Dancing resonates deep within us, and it is something that comes oh-so-naturally. For instance, babies, dance! They do not consciously dance or even know they're dancing, but the way they let their limbs move freely about, waving in and around the light, is a most primal form of dancing.

Dancing makes us feel powerful, and when we feel powerful, we feel good. Our heart gets a great workout, we increase circulation, release endorphins, and thoroughly energize ourselves. And when we dance, we let go. We unknot, unfurl, and disengage our brains, letting our bodies take over.

Dance can be incredibly therapeutic. Why, there are even dance therapy organizations. Dance therapy uses expressive movement as a healing tool for both personal expression and psychological or emotional wellness. Practitioners work with people with physical disabilities, addiction issues, sexual abuse histories, eating disorders, and other concerns.

We all know of the more traditional and contemporary types of dance—the waltz, foxtrot, polka, rumba, ballet, funky jazz—but you should also familiarize yourself with some alternative dance forms. I've been known to attend a trance dance on occasion. This is one of the most primordial ways to move the body, free the mind, and connect with spirit. Shamans and indigenous peoples have practiced trance dancing for thousands of years. This ancient transformative and healing technique is becoming quite popular. Have a trance dance evening in your salon/spa. I dare you!

Anyone can dance. Just like the Sufi whirling dervishes, you swirl, twirl, chant, and channel as you dance your way to ecstasy. Turn on your favorite music, close your eyes, and let your spirit move you.

How to Trance Dance

These wonderful trance dance instructions come from the Natale Institute.

The most important advice related to Trance Dance is to trust the process. Let the process reveal experiences beyond the limits of time and space. Also, Trance Dance does not require a great deal of space, since the dance largely happens within.

Turn on your musical selection—one that allows you to tune in to the rhythm and move freely. Stand with your feet parallel to your shoulders and let your body and mind relax.

Close your eyes, or preferably wear a bandanna or a blindfold over them, so that your eyes only see the vast inner landscape of your consciousness.

Become aware of your breathing. Inhale and exhale deeply, filling your lungs entirely. Do this for 3 to 5 minutes. This will awaken your energizer within.

Relax and allow your body to move to the rhythm. Soon you will feel a vibration or energy moving through your body. At this point, you the dancer will disappear and become the dance. The energizer within will awaken, and you will experience profound emotions and a peaceful connection to your own immortality.

This entire process will take between 30 and 45 minutes.

When the music ends, take 5 to 15 minutes to be still and integrate your experiences.

Movement Therapy

Similar to dance in terms of benefits but definitely more systematized are several organized movement therapies with highly regarded reputations for their ability to initiate mindbody healing. The most well-known disciplines are yoga, Pilates, and tai chi, but many other movement therapies exist. Practitioners lead their clients through movements, body-awareness techniques, and/or breathing exercises designed to expand awareness and improve health. These techniques serve to replace old, habitual body movement patterns with healthy behavior.

If you feel that the way you hold your body while working is less than desirable, whether due to bad habits, past accidents, physical traumas, or emotional issues, and that you are thus creating unnatural patterns of rigidity, consider any of these therapies. As you read through the following list, remember, it is not all-inclusive, but rather covers the better-known approaches.

Alexander Technique—Practitioners, using gentle hands-on guidance and verbal instruction, teach simple, efficient ways of moving that ultimately improve balance, posture, and coordination while simultaneously relieving tension and pain.

Feldenkrais Method—This method combines movement training, gentle touch, and verbal dialogue to help create freer, more efficient movement. Feldenkrais takes two forms: In individual hands-on sessions (Functional Integration), the practitioner's touch is used to address the student's breathing and body alignment. In a series of slow, nonaerobic motions (Awareness Through Movement), students learn improved ways to move the body. The Method is frequently used to treat stress and tension, to prevent recurring injuries, and to help improve balance and coordination.

Hellerwork—This technique combines deep-tissue muscle therapy and movement education with dialogue about the emotional issues that may underlie physical posture. Participants go through eleven 60-to-90-minute sessions. Stressing the mindbody connection, Hellerwork treats chronic pain and helps healthy people learn to live more comfortably in their bodies.

Qi Gong (Chi-Kung)—This ancient Chinese exercise system aims to stimulate and balance the flow of qi (chi), or vital energy, along the acupuncture meridians, or energy pathways. Qi Gong is used to reduce stress, improve blood circulation, enhance immune function, and treat a variety of medical conditions.

Ohashiatsu—This system of physical techniques, exercise, and meditation is used to relieve tension and fatigue and induce a sense of harmony and peace. The practitioner first assesses a person's state by feeling the hara (the area below the navel). Then, using continuous and flowing movements, the practitioner presses and stretches the body's energy channels, working in unison with the person's breathing.

Ortho-Bionomy—This therapy involves the use of noninvasive, gentle touch along with dialogue and instruction in common movements such as walking, sitting, standing, and reaching. Practitioners may work with the energy field surrounding the person. The goal here is to enhance well-being and empowerment, as opposed to physical healing per se.

Pilates—This is a whole-body workout. Very balancing! It is aerobic, flexibility, and strengthening movement all rolled into one. It is a system that includes several hundred controlled, precise movements done on one of seven pieces of equipment along with extensive mat work. It is aimed at stretching and strengthening back, buttocks, and abdomenal muscles. Most always, the emphasis is on form, along with intense concentration and coordinated breathing.

Rosen Method—This method combines gentle touch and verbal communication to evoke relaxation and self-awareness. Because the work can bring up buried feelings and memories, it is sometimes used as a tool for personal growth as well as pain relief.

Rubenfield Synergy Method—This movement therapy uses gentle touch, movement, verbal exchange, and the imagination to access memories and emotions locked in the body. The approach, developed by healer Ilana Rubenfield, integrates elements of the Alexander Technique, the Feldenkrais Method, Gestalt therapy, and hypnotherapy. Because it combines bodywork and psychotherapy, this method may be used for specific physical or emotional problems or for personal growth.

Tai chi—This is actually a martial art, practiced to improve physical fitness and promote mental and spiritual development. The highly controlled movements within the various Tai chi forms or disciplines are thought to unite body and mind and bring balance to an individual's life. Tai chi is also used in combination with other therapies as a treatment for back problems, ulcers, and stress.

Trager Bodywork—This approach seeks to address the mental roots of muscle tension. By gently rocking, cradling, and moving the student's body, the practitioner encourages the student to see how physically restrictive patterns can be changed. Trager bodywork is meant to promote relaxation and increase mobility and mental clarity. It is used by athletes for performance enhancement and by those with musculoskeletal and back problems.

Think Your Way to a Better Body

When you work out from within, the power of the mindbody connection can help you build muscle and lose fat. The results may amaze you. Try to wean yourself off walking the treadmill or spinning the bike to blaring music or mindless television. And for goodness sake, never, ever do yoga to television (unless of course, you're working with a video or specific yoga TV show)! You really don't want to distract your mind from the magnificence of everything going on inside your body while practicing any form of physical activity. It is so important to remember that physical activity is not something to get through; it is something to blissfully enjoy. It's all in your perception of the experience. Pay attention to your breath and to every sensation. Visualize your body performing at its best. This kind of focus and attitude has been proven to greatly enhance the benefits of an exercise session, whether you're golfing, biking, practicing tai chi, or pumping iron.

See the Light of Day

Most of the therapies we've discussed are done indoors, but you should also remember the importance of taking yourself outdoors occasionally. Try to get outside at least once a day. Walk in the natural light, enjoy the sights, sounds, and smells. Wake up to the extraordinary beauty around you! This will disengage you from the world of machines, and as you expose yourself to the sun, sky, and wind, take time to thank Mother Earth for all she does to nurture us.

On a slightly more scientific level, the natural "light clock" activated when sunlight enters your eyes influences your body's master glands, specifically affecting sleeping and waking cycles, hormone secretion, growth, sexual maturation, body temperature, appetite, and moods and behavior. Natural light is also needed for the metabolization of vitamin D, the sunshine vitamin, through your skin. This vitamin's primary function is to stimulate the absorption of calcium, so for your bones' sake, let the sunshine in.

Ergonomics

Ergonomics is about maximizing productivity by minimizing bodily fatigue and discomfort. In other words, you want to end the day feeling as great as you did when you started—well, almost as great. Some fatigue is only natural. Discomfort, however, is not.

If you control stress (Chapter Four), get your nourishment (Chapter Six), remain physically fit (I think I made my point on that subject in this chapter!), and work in an ergonomically sound environment, you should be as energetically and creatively present for your 9 A.M. appointment as you are for your 5 P.M. appointment. (Note to all fellow beauty pros: When it comes to controlling stress, take control of your schedule, and do not book beyond your physical capabilities. No amount of attention to stress control, ergonomics, nutrition, or physical fitness will combat irrational, impossible workloads!)

Many of you may already be familiar with ergonomics—the science of interacting safely and efficiently with the objects in your work environment. Maybe you call this body mechanics. If you are not yet acquainted with the wonders of this concept, the first rule is to remember this very important maxim: fit your job to your body, and not your body to your job. Yes, I realize that in many cases this is easier said than done, but it's worth every effort. Once you understand the importance of shifting your patterns of movement to those that are most ergonomically correct, you will be in a much better position to love your calling.

Hand and wrist motions, reaching up, reaching out, bending over, twisting, standing, sitting—all these movements are quite natural. But if you do them a hundred times a day, and always incorrectly, you could be setting yourself up for some serious physiological problems. These problems can become restrictive.

As beauty professionals, we may be required to compromise our bodies in a variety of ways. You may stand all day in a small area or hold your body in unnatural positions for protracted periods of time. You may need to bend your head and neck too far forward or sideways for lengths of time, elevate your arms for too long, assume awkward hand and finger positions, or lean forward too often from the lower back or waist. Contracting your muscles in these ways could lead to chronic or cumulative trauma disorders (CTDs). These disorders may include but are not limited to tendinitis, carpal tunnel syndrome, thoracic outlet syndrome, bursitis, varicose veins, pinched nerves or sciatica, and ruptured or herniated discs.

Now, I know that all of this sounds very unromantic and unpoetic—especially for those of us who became a beauty professional because of the creativity, self-expression, and artistic voice it affords us. However, too many beauty professionals leave our wonderful profession because of debilitating conditions brought on by the physicality of our work. It doesn't need to be this way. So bear with me for the brief bit of information that follows. It could very well open your eyes and mind to some specific movements that may be the underlying cause of your own aches and pains.

Name That Pain

Tendinitis: Tendons attach muscles to bone, and when you use (or overuse) your hands, wrists, and/or shoulders, this can cause the tendons to become swollen and inflamed. Over time, this stress can bring on tendinitis, making it painful to use your hand, especially when grasping things. Inflamed, painful shoulders can make it difficult to raise your arms.

Carpal Tunnel Syndrome: The carpal tunnel, in the wrist, is a structure through which a nerve and several tendons pass. If the tendons in this tunnel swell due to incorrect usage or overuse, the nerve is squeezed. Numbness, tingling, and weakness in the hand are signs of carpal tunnel syndrome.

Thoracic Outlet Syndrome: A common affliction among beauty professionals, this is a constriction of the nerves and blood vessels to the arms. It most often occurs when you raise your shoulders up toward your ears while also raising your arms, or, more precisely, when you shrug your shoulders as you raise your arms. Instead, you want to raise your arms by using the shoulder joint, keeping the shoulders relaxed and in a natural position. Numbness, tingling, swelling, and coldness may be signs of thoracic outlet syndrome.

Bursitis: Bursa are fluid-filled sacs located between the tendons and bones in the shoulder. When squeezed excessively between the tendons and bones, the bursa become inflamed, causing bursitis. Bursitis can make it painful, if not impossible, to raise your arm. Often holding your arms out away from the body, or frequently holding them above shoulder height, can lead to this problem.

Pinched Nerves or Sciatica: When standing in a normal posture, there is a small hollow in the back of the neck as well as the back. When you bend forward, the discs between the vertebrae of your spine are squeezed. When this happens, the discs can press against—or pinch—different parts of the spine, including nerves. If this bending occurs constantly, it can cause pain in the neck and back as well as pain or numbness in the arms and legs. Twisting excessively can also cause similar problems.

Ruptured or Herniated Discs: If you spend many years bending forward incorrectly and/or twisting excessively, squeezing the discs along the spine, the jelly-like substance inside each disc might begin to leak out. If a large quantity leaks out all at once, we say that the disc is ruptured or herniated. This problem can have serious consequences, including excessive pain, numbness, or even an inability to move. This requires immediate medical attention.

Varicose Veins: Long periods of standing can produce varicose or swollen veins. This is a sign that the blood circulation in your legs is not working as efficiently as possible.

The Path Toward Prevention

Prevention is obviously the key to alleviating the problems I have just outlined. Again, it is very important that you fit the job to yourself, and not fit yourself to the job. This all boils down to keeping your body's posture and alignment in the most healthful position for you. Mindfulness of the postures, movements, and positions that you use, coupled with your choice of tools and equipment, can greatly affect your comfort and the health of your musculoskeletal system, specifically the hands, wrists, shoulders, neck, back, feet, and legs. Always remember: if something doesn't feel right, or if you are feeling tremendous bodily fatigue or specific pains over the course of the day, then chances are there is probably a more efficient and ergonomically correct way in which to use your body.

I also recommend that you begin doing some sort of regular stretching routine or yoga session before heading off to work. Think of this as a warm-up for you, the beauty athlete. Don't forget to take those stretch breaks in between clients. As you stretch, counterpose any posture that you may have been holding for an extended period, and remember to breathe deeply as you do your stretches. Flex or harmony balls, used during rest periods or even at home, will strengthen and condition the muscles and joints in your hands and forearms. You might also learn to incorporate mini-pauses into your work flow. Let your arms drop down by your sides. Roll your shoulders. Stand tall. All the while, breathe deeply and slowly. Now move smoothly into the next action. This is not a break, and no one will even notice—except you, of course!

Naturally, controlling stress is an integral part of enhancing physical comfort, as is overall physical fitness. Regular cardiovascular, flexibility, and strengthening exercises go a long way toward preventing aches, strains, and pain.

Reflect on and describe your physical movements over the course of your workday. Include the variety and intensity of the activities that you perform, and the involvement of your body. For instance, when you cut hair, do you concentrate on keeping your wrist in a neutral or straight position as much as possible? When you give a massage, do you concentrate on avoiding hyperextending your thumb? When you give manicures, do you concentrate on bending forward from the hips and keeping your knuckles below your wrists?

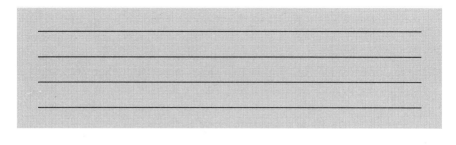

Move This Way

Here's a quick list to help you evaluate whether you are presently using healthful motions. Try to alter any stressful patterns:

- Try to keep your wrists as straight as possible. Evaluate your motions and change any technique that has you constantly bending your wrists up (extension), down (flexion), or from side to side. You are most likely to assume these unhealthy positions when cutting hair, holding the hair dryer, using a round brush, giving a manicure, or providing a massage. Roll the handle of the round brush between the fingers, as opposed to using backward and forward wrist motions.
- Avoid repeated forceful gripping or pinching motions. Make sure your scissors fit your hand and are sharp, lubricated, and balanced. Select a curling iron with a handle that revolves. Be mindful of these motions when performing massages.
- Avoid excessive thumb drilling in massage—it can cause damage to the synovial membrane in the thumb joint.
- Try to avoid holding your arms out away from your body while working, or holding your elbows above your shoulders for extended time periods. These postures can produce shoulder strain. Adjust the height of your workstation chair or massage table, putting yourself closer to the client. Swivel the chair as often as needed so you do not overextend your reach. Adjust your work flow to decrease the amount of time your arms are held at angles of 60 degrees or higher. Consider holding the hair dryer sideways to avoid raising your arms above shoulder level excessively. And remember those mini-pauses.
- Be mindful of how you bend, twist, and reach. Done incorrectly or in a frantic hurry, these motions can result in neck and back strain. Try to keep your elbows by your side whenever possible, and try to keep your back straight. Bend from the hips or in the knees as opposed to from the waist.

- Invest in well-fitting shoes that provide good arch support. Consider rubber-soled shoes, and possibly shock-absorbing and/or orthopedic inserts. Foot and leg problems often stem from wearing improper or uncomfortable shoes, especially when standing for long periods on hard floors. Above all else, do not wear high heels! Heels displace your center of gravity, and protecting this center of gravity is integral to body wellness.
- Stand on a cushioned foot mat. It's incredible what a difference this makes, as it helps prevent or reduce fatigue.
- Work with your shoulders down, and let a whole lot of muscles share the load. Shoulders up around the ears are sometimes called the shoulder hanger syndrome. The name is funny, but the pain it produces is not.
- Place one foot on a small stool when standing for long periods. This will help change the angle of the curve in your lower back, and thus reduce muscular tension. Or if salon conditions permit, alternate between sitting on a stool and standing.
- Gently tilt the client's head as needed for your comfort.
- In massage, work from your center and do not lean into the table. Put the force of your whole body into a stroke, as opposed to just using your thumbs, hands, arms, shoulder, or back. Brace the thumb with the other thumb, hand, or elbow, giving extra strength and support. When possible brace the hands together, so that the thumbs support each other. Use the thumb as a sensor, then use a stronger body part, like the elbow, to exert pressure. Use the mound right under the thumb when working on legs and arms. Be careful not to compress the wrist.
- When manicuring, have the client extend her hand toward you, instead of you reaching across. This helps avoid tension in your arms, hands, and shoulders.

Now that you have a better idea how to move your body in a healthy way, let's talk a bit about the equipment you use.

- Evaluate your work-station design. Well-designed stations and equipment allow you to keep your wrists, shoulders, neck, and back in the most healthful positions.
- Work stations should have ample space between them, so you can move freely and keep roll-abouts close by.
- Cabinets should be within easy reach.

- Freestanding shampoo bowls are best, since they allow you to do the job from behind instead of from the side. Working from the side forces the shampooer to use unnatural twists, bends, and reaches, which can create or aggravate back problems.
- Hydraulic chairs are okay, allowing you to make adjustments up and down within five or six inches. Electrical chairs are better, usually with a broader range of adjustment than hydraulic chairs.
- Rolling stools let you sit while working. Those with a wide, bicycle-type seat are ideal.
- Manicure tables with armrests are better for the beauty pro as well as the client. If no armrests are available, folded towels can help support the arms. This helps keep the wrists in a more neutral position while you are working.
- Facialists' chairs should adjust up to 36 inches.
- For facialists and manicurists, consider chairs that tilt forward, or use a wedge-shaped cushion in order to let the chair do the bending for you. This allows you to lean forward at the hips without bending the spine.

Some final reminders:

- Take control of your schedule, and never book beyond your physical capabilities.
- Do simple stretches over the course of the day.
- Take mini-breaks, or use pauses creatively to bring the head back over the shoulders, stand up tall, bring the chin in, breathe, and then flow into the next movement.
- Improve your overall physical fitness in order to significantly reduce injury risks.
- Take up leisure-time activities that use different actions and postures than those used during your workday.
- Respect your most valuable tool: your body, as guided by your mind. From a higher level of consciousness, the mindbody physiology strives toward its highest good. If your body is unable and unwilling, there is probably a deep chasm between the mind and the body. You've heard that saying, "the mind is willing, but the body is unable." This deep chasm can be repaired by approaching every action that you take with the utmost mindfulness.
- Make every beautifying ritual with every client a thing of beauty. Move with your body relaxed and never rigid. Work toward fluidity in all your movements. Anything we do as beauty professionals should indeed be poetry in motion—like a beautiful dance.

Simply Yoga

I invite you to become familiar with these simple stretches, all easily incorporated into your workday. Don't let their simplicity fool you, though, for each posture is incredibly rejuvenating.

Do these one at a time or in combination: it all depends on what part of your body needs TLC, and also how much time you have in-between clients. Try to do counterposes to positions that you consistently hold your body in as you work. And definitely try to do the modified shoulder stand with a chair or against a wall at least once partway through your day. Remember to breathe smoothly and fluidly while performing these postures, and pay attention to every sensation in your body. Feel the stretch.

Modified Shoulder Stand

This powerful restorative pose leaves you feeling refreshed and reinvigorated. It can reduce stress and fatigue, release muscular tension, improve sleep, lower blood pressure, enhance immune response, manage chronic pain, strengthen the respiratory system and circulation, slow down your breathing and resting heartbeat rates, and lead the body to a state in which the nervous system and the mind naturally relax. It gives the body a respite from the unrelenting force of gravity exerted on it, reversing the vascular flow of blood to the heart. It can also bring a rich supply of nutrients to the spine and possibly relieve varicose veins.

The legs may be placed on a chair or up against a wall. Be careful to keep your knees relaxed and not to lock the knee joints into a rigid position. The backs of the hips should rest comfortably on the ground. You can also opt to place a pillow under the buttocks. This will tilt the pelvis upward slightly, accentuating the flow of blood to the upper torso. With your arms by your sides, roll your shoulders under so the shoulder blades lie flat. Place your elbows beside your body. Push the elbows and the head back flat. Feel the chest lift slightly, and draw the shoulder blades

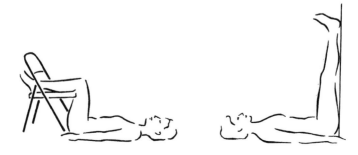

down toward the waist. Extend the back of the neck. Drop the belly and relax, opening the heart and lungs. Continue for as long as time permits. This feels so good if you've been on your feet for awhile and if you've been curling everything in and forward.

Neck and Shoulder Stretches

The neck and shoulders are particularly vulnerable to tension and stress. These stretches can profoundly release stress and built-up tension in these muscles. These stretches can prevent chronic neck and shoulder pain when practiced regularly, and they allow for greater blood flow to the brain. They also promote calm, clear thinking. Do each one of these stretches while breathing naturally and smoothly. Hold for as long as comfortable, or as time permits. Counter with a stretch toward the opposite side where applicable.

Bowing Forward
Standing or sitting straight, with both feet flat on the floor, gently float your head to your chest. Feel the wonderful stretch along the back of the neck and shoulders.

Ear to Shoulder

With spine straight and feet flat on floor, gently roll the right ear down toward the shoulder. Release any tension that you feel and breathe. Gently come back upward. Repeat to the other side.

Head Side to Side

Sitting straight, turn your head to the side as far as is comfortable. Try to look toward the wall behind you. Repeat to the opposite side.

Shoulder Shrugs
Sitting or standing up straight, on the inhale, raise your shoulders up toward the ears. Now on the exhale, thoroughly release the shoulders downward as far as they'll go. Feel the release of held tension in this area.

Shoulder Rolls
With the spine straight, stand with both feet flat on the floor and arms relaxed by your sides. Roll the shoulders in a circular fashion, moving upward and back. Repeat several times. Then repeat moving forward.

Hands Clasped Behind Head

Clasp your hands behind your head (so they are resting on occipital). Gently flex your elbows back, with the upper shoulders flexed inward. This can dispel tension in the upper shoulders and back.

Elbow Pull

Place the right hand on the left shoulder. Place the other hand on the elbow of the right arm and pull the right elbow in toward the chest. Don't raise the shoulder. The left arm is doing the work. This stretches and elongates the upper arm and definitely unkinks the shoulder area. Do on the other side.

Arm Against Wall

Stretch one arm straight back at shoulder height and press it full length, from shoulder to hand, against a wall. Keep the palm flat against the wall. The arm should be at shoulder height. Rest your hip against the wall. Breathe smoothly and fluidly. Bring the shoulder that's not against the wall back and away from the wall as far as comfortably possible, while keeping the other shoulder against the wall. Take several breaths, then release. Repeat on the other side. There should not be any pain in this stretch! For more stretch, you can try taking your hand a little higher on the wall.

Hands Clasped in Front

With spine straight and both feet flat on the floor, stretch your arms out in front of your heart center, or chest. Shoulders are relaxed, fingers interlaced, palms stretched outward. Reach out with your arms and hands, keeping your back straight. Breathe smoothly and fluidly. Gently bring your arms back down into the prayer pose (see page 129) or down to the side. You can move from this pose directly into the Overhead Stretch if you like.

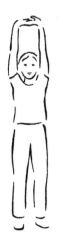

Overhead Stretch

This stretch loosens your upper-body muscles. While seated or standing, inhale and raise your arms overhead. As you exhale, twist your wrists and turn your palms upward. Keep your hands in this position throughout the stretch. On the next inhalation, stretch your arms upward as far as you can reach. Imagine your arms originating from your waist rather than your shoulders. Press your palms toward the ceiling. Relax as you exhale.

Side Stretch

You can go from the Overhead Stretch directly into the Side Stretch, or do it as a separate stretch. This stretch relaxes shoulder muscles while serving to improve circulation and digestion. Stand with your entire back against a wall, feet about six inches apart. Inhale as you raise your arms overhead, hands interlaced and palms facing upward. Exhale while stretching the upraised arms toward the left, keeping shoulders and hips against the wall. Feel the stretch along the entire right side off the body. Breathe! Straighten on an inhalation. Repeat on the other side.

Hand and Wrist Poses

These postures stretch the hands, fingers, wrists, and arms. They lengthen the armpits and stimulate the lymph system. They lengthen the spine, and they balance the entire physiology.

Prayer Pose

With the spine straight and feet flat on the floor, place your hands together, finger to finger, palm to palm, in a prayer pose in front of your heart. As you inhale slowly, press the palms firmly together, fingers pointing up. Holding the prayer pose, exhale slowly as you lower the hands as far as possible. Inhale and slowly lift the hands in front of the heart center. Repeat several times.

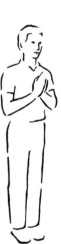

Wrist Stretch and Palm Stretch

These stretches are particularly helpful in preventing or easing tendinitis. Remember to see your doctor if you have recurring wrist problems. Be gentle with your wrists. Overstretching can make matters worse instead of better.

Wrist Stretch

This stretch stimulates blood flow to the wrist area and increases flexibility. It also lengthens the muscles and tendons. Sitting close to your work station or any tabletop, place your right elbow on a flat, hard surface, with your palm up. Let the weight of your left arm rest in the fingers of the right hand, gently stretching the right wrist. Allow the weight of the left arm, assisted by gravity, to gently stretch the wrist. Hold for a few breaths. When done, gently bend the wrist in the opposite direction to counteract the backward bend. Repeat with the opposite wrist. Try to do this at intervals throughout the day.

Palm Stretch

This stretch opens up the wrist by stretching the palm area and relieving held tensions. Place your right elbow on a table or your station, palm facing up. Bend the wrist gently back by letting your left hand hang from the right thumb. Hold for a few breaths. When done, gently bend the wrist in the opposite direction to counteract the backward bend. Repeat with the other wrist.

Seated Forward Bend

Whether done from a standing position or seated, this exercise stretches every muscle from the top of the head to the back of the heels. Sit toward the front half of your chair, feet flat on the floor about hip-width apart. On the inhale, stretch your arms upward over your head. As you are exhaling, bend forward as far as your body comfortably wants to go. Rest your torso on top of your thighs if possible. Your arms may be 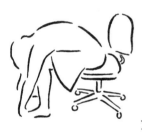 touching the floor or resting at some point along your legs. As you breathe smoothly and fluidly, feel yourself sinking farther into the pose. When you are ready to come upward, place your hands on your knees and slowly come upward, one vertebra at a time, until you are in an upright position. Rest here for a moment, paying attention to the sensations in your body.

Backbend

This eases tension in the upper and lower back and expands the chest cavity. Stand with your back to the wall, feet about a foot from the wall, hip-width apart and parallel. Raise your arms overhead and place your palms against the wall, fingers pointing down. Exhale and evenly arch your spine forward, pressing your hip bones forward and lifting your chest. Direct your gaze upward. Hold for a few breaths and release on an exhalation.

Seated Spinal Twist

This stretch is rejuvenating for the spine, lengthening it and enhancing blood flow and flexibility. Since we beauty professionals frequently use our side-to-side range of motion, you will find this stretch particularly good for strengthening and toning the spine. Sit straight, cross the right leg over the left leg, and place your left hand on your right knee, all the while breathing smoothly. Inhale and lengthen upward. As you are exhaling, simultaneously place your right hand around the back of your chair and gently twist your head and spine around to the right, looking over the right shoulder. Breathe smoothly and hold this position as long as you comfortably can. Inhale, then release, coming back to center. Repeat on the other side.

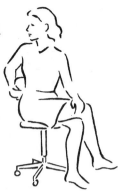

Cat's Pose

This is actually two poses, moving from the dog into the cat. This combination stretch increases the spine's flexibility. Stand with your legs about hip-width apart and your hands on your work station or on a stable chair. As you inhale, you want to move the spine up and out. Do this by tilting the tailbone and pelvis up, letting the spine curve up and out, dropping the stomach low, and lifting your head up. Stretch gently and breathe. As you exhale, proceed into the cat by moving the spine inward. Do this by reversing the spinal bend, tilting the pelvis downward, drawing the spine upward, and pulling the chest and stomach in. Repeat several times. Hold each posture as long as desired.

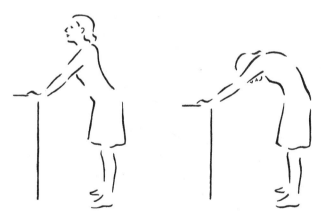

Child's Pose

A rejuvenating posture, this stretch is tremendously nurturing. In a seated position, place both feet flat on the floor, ankles and knees together. Place your arms behind your back with one hand resting inside the other. Gently come forward until your chest is resting on your knees. Breathe smoothly and fluidly. There should be no strain. As an option, you may also place your arms on your knees and rest your head on them. Release any tension that you feel in your body. Now place your hands on your knees and slowly push upward, supporting your lower back. Relax for a few moments with your hands in your lap.

Remember to breathe and honor your body. I recommend that these postures be practiced in flat or low-heeled shoes or in bare feet. Heels shift the spinal alignment of the body into unnatural positions that could prevent you from realizing the full benefit of certain stretches. Don't go any further than your mindbody physiology wants to go. Use any of these stretches over the course of the day to maintain high energy levels and help stave off muscular aches, pains, and tensions. Enjoy!

These stretches are not intended as a replacement for qualified medical care. If you experience any health issues with your body, see a physician before engaging in this or any form of physical activity. In particular, pregnant women and persons with any form of cardiovascular disease are urged to confer with their doctor.

Notes:

Chapter Six

Nourishing Wisdom

> " Tell me what you eat, and
> I will tell you what you are. "
>
> *Anthelme Brillat-Savarin*

Truly, we experience some of life's greatest pleasures through our sense of taste. Yes, we consume food for nourishment, but eating also brings us a veritable buffet of additional pleasures.

For many of us, meals provide a nurturing and blissful way to connect with others. On the surface, eating becomes an activity. On a much deeper level, it is the way many of us sustain human relationships. Whether it's two friends sharing lunch, an entire village feasting in celebration, pals meeting for food and drink, extended families reuniting, or business associates sealing a deal over breakfast, we often connect with others via the activity of eating.

In addition, food represents an outer expression of our spirituality. This includes bread and wine at a Christian communion, unleavened bread 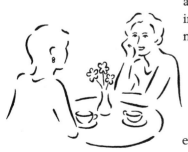 and herbs at the Jewish Passover, harvest offerings in traditional Native American ceremonies, and bountiful spreads enjoyed by many cultures at life-altering events such as births, weddings, and deaths. Even during life's more private spiritual moments, food can serve to nourish the soul. A simple snack or meal can intensify romantic interludes, encourage fabulous connection, fuel flirtatious

> **"Let** food be your medicine, and medicine be your food. **"**

Hippocrates

energy, bring into focus great good fortune in life, and ultimately provide a host of additional potentially sensual or enlightening experiences.

Indeed, food may also become a metaphor. So many of us overindulge in unhealthy types or quantities of food, desperately hoping to feed a deep spiritual hunger. Grossly oversimplified, anorexia, an act of self-starvation, is often triggered by a need to gain control of one's life; obesity may result when one forgets to feed one's heart with love and attempts to fill the resulting void with junk food binges. Starving souls, whether famished for things or experiences, will always seek to fill up somehow.

In this chapter, we will examine all four uses for food—nourishment, human connection, spirituality, and misplaced dependence on food to feed the soul. As you continue reading, remember that knowledge is power. Learn as much as you can about how food affects you. Remember that you are the ultimate choice maker when it comes to what you will or will not eat. As you learn to eat with love and awareness, visualize how food is nourishing both your mind and body. Let this be your focus every time you take a bite—whether it's a tiny snack or a great feast. Your life will be transformed.

A Good Argument for Good Nutrition

I've been there. Just like many of you. I used to go into the salon dispensary and down a fast-food burger—everything on it—coupled with fries and the obligatory diet cola. More often than not, I hurriedly gulped while standing—a big no-no, terrible for digestion. But this was a lifetime ago for me. Seeing how an unhealthy diet began to negatively affect my performance, looks, and physical wellness, I chose to educate myself about healthy eating habits. This choice will ultimately give me a chance to live a longer and more vibrant life.

My food choices serve to advance the flow of life-force energy through my body. Eating a balanced diet of nutritious organic and whole foods gives me tremendous energy, a strong, resilient body, and greater immunity to emotional as well as physical toxins. By selecting foods that fortify my arteries and veins, I am more able to absorb and use nutrients. Every cell in my body is working in physiological harmony, doing the right job—clearing the way for glowing skin, shiny lustrous hair, strong nails, and radiant eyes. How's this for a dynamic daily positive affirmation and creative visualization?

Before we get into specific food choices, though, I urge everyone to make a conscious decision to eat healthfully—and routinely. Yes, that's right. We Americans regularly disrupt our biological rhythms by not creating a routine for healthful eating. We forget or simply do not make time to sit down and eat three square meals a day. Every day all of us should have a minimum of three balanced meals of nutrient-dense, fiber-rich foods—foods that keep your blood sugar stable and give your body a steady source of energy. This is of paramount importance for us beauty pros. Standing on your feet all day, interacting with a variety of personality types (associates as well as clients), working within a tightly packed schedule, connecting with various environmental and emotional toxins—all these stressors can deplete our energy levels and exacerbate free-radical formation in our mindbody physiology, among other things. If you try to run your body all day on a cup of coffee or orange juice for breakfast and a yogurt or hot dog for lunch, you will run out of energy. This chapter will serve as a useful primer on nutritional awareness—an awareness that is an important part of your career consciousness. And as you become more adept in the basics of good nutrition, you will want to share this type of information with fellow beauty professionals as well as clients.

Clean Up Your Eating Habits

When I say each one of us should choose nutritious organic and whole foods, this implies clean food—and no, I am not referring to food washed with one of those new oh-so-handy nontoxic cleansers. Clean food refers to food free of pesticide residues, antibiotics, growth hormones, genetically modified organisms, artificial preservatives, flavoring, and coloring, and irradiation. Irradiation involves nuclear waste energy used to eradicate bacteria like E. coli or salmonella; while this process does destroy bacteria, it also changes a food's molecular structure and creates high levels of free radicals. Clean food also retains maximum nutritional value through proper processing, packaging, transportation, and storage.

If you offer only clean foods and beverages in your salon or spa, tell the world. Put this information in your advertisements, on a small placard hanging by the reception desk, and in your establishment's front window. A growing number of people are seeking out these kinds of environments, and you may end up boosting your business as well as your clients' energy levels.

The Great Supplement Debate

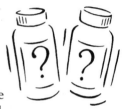

Another choice that you want to consider concerns supplements—a.k.a. vitamins. If you eat a well-balanced, organic, whole-foods diet, you most likely give your body an ample amount of vitamins, minerals, and antioxidants. Still, some nutritionists say that even the most carefully chosen diet still needs a bit of boosting. These experts insist that the overall quality of our food generally lowers the amount of vitamins, minerals, trace minerals, amino acids, essential fatty acids, and enzymes available, thus making it mandatory to take a high-quality multivitamin and mineral supplement and possibly supplemental antioxidants as well. If you are unsure which side of the fence you are on, ask for guidance from a professional nutritionist or your primary-care physician.

If you do decide to take supplements, be sure to read the label and identify whether your supplement is synthesized or not. The body is ill-equipped to metabolize synthesized supplements, so you may very well be wasting your money. Lyophilized supplements are in liquid form and more readily absorbed. There are also nonsynthetic tablet supplements made from whole food derivatives.

I can't emphasize enough how valuable a visit with a nutritionist can be. Whether you are looking to intelligently shift your eating habits or select the right supplements, nutritional counseling will prove quite transformative and educational. Look for nutritionists who team up with medical doctors. This may help consultations run more smoothly and speedily. Also, teaming up with a physician gives the nutrition expert an opportunity to request specific state-of-the-art diagnostic tests. In addition, you want to be careful about selecting a reputable nutritionist. Ask about credentials and training. Recommendations are great, too.

The Flavor of Life

It's a fact. The American diet is top-heavy in saturated fats, sugars, salts, and cholesterol. More then ever, we eat fast food. These quick meals are typically made with excessive amounts of fat and hydrogenated oils containing transfatty acids—ingredients that weaken the integrity of our cells and set the stage for certain cancers and heart disease. And for those of you who think the high fiber content in a super-duper burger with fries counts, forget it. In order for you to benefit from the cancer-fighting properties that fiber provides (particularly when it comes to colon cancer), it has to be something like fresh veggies and fruits!

Ours is a society that is always on the go, but our diet may very well be stopping us dead in our tracks. I saw a very effective American Heart Association ad. It said, "What to eat if you don't like hospital food. Fresh vegetables and fruits, whole grains, low-fat dairy products, lean meat, poultry, and fish. That's the kind of diet that may keep you away from the cardiac intensive care unit. Exercise is another way to reduce your risk of heart disease and stroke." Pretty effective copy, huh?

So I urge you to begin fighting the urge to consume massive amounts of fats, sugar, and salt today. Teach yourself to truly relish the delicious natural flavors of life. Eat a fresh carrot and savor the sublime sweetness. Try your whole-grain cereal without added sugar and appreciate the grain's natural sweetness. Eat your watermelon without salt, and your grapefruit without sugar. And cut back on the dressing over your salad or butter over your steamed veggies. Instead of saturated fat from butter, dribble on a bit of organic olive, peanut, or sesame oil. Infuse these oils with herbs and spices. In fact, instead of reaching for the salt or sugar, use herbs and spices in all your favorite foods. Really taste the fresh, delectable, pungent flavors. Your taste buds will thank you!

Think about your eating habits. Reflect and see them clearly for what they really are. Consider a typical day at work as well as a typical day off.

How many meals do you eat?

How many of these meals are eaten outside the home?

Do you snack a great deal?

What sorts of snacks do you eat?

Do you try to have protein, carbohydrates, and good fats at every meal?

Do you carefully plan and prepare meals to take to work?

Do you cook meals from scratch?

Do you buy precooked meals?

Do you know how to read boxed, canned, and bagged food labels?

Do you purchase certified organic foods?

How often do you add sugar, salt, or butter to your foods?

How often do you use fresh herbs and spices?

Do you need to give your typical daily menu a little TLC? Jot down a few ways to achieve better eating habits.

_____

_____

_____

_____

_____

_____

_____

_____

Make a grocery shopping list that supports your resolutions to eat better.

_____

_____

_____

_____

_____

_____

_____

The Nitty-Gritty on Nutrients

Our wellness depends on getting the proper supply of nutrients. Nutrients are the basic components of food, and, generally speaking, they serve three functions:

- to provide fuel for energy
- to provide the raw material necessary for our body tissues and organs to renew and repair themselves
- to regulate our bodies' ongoing metabolic functions

There are forty specific nutrients in our food, and these nutrients fall into the following categories: carbohydrates, proteins, fats, and water. All the vitamins and minerals we need can be found within these categories, especially when eating a balanced diet of whole, organic, clean food.

The Caloric Nutrients

Carbohydrates, found in whole grains, vegetables, and fruits, should account for 40 to 50 percent of your daily nutrient intake. Through these vital foods we optimize energy levels, get the fiber necessary to regulate digestion and absorb nutrients, regulate cholesterol levels, and promote healthy bowel function. As it binds to cholesterol and aids in elimination, fiber allows for an uninterrupted flow of nutrients to the entire body.

Proteins are the body's building blocks. The brain, muscles, skin, hair, and connective tissue are all composed primarily of protein. Protein is also needed for the body to produce enzymes and hormones. Protein should comprise approximately 20 to 30 percent of your daily diet, and it is important to choose proteins low in cholesterol and saturated fat. Some examples are animal foods such as lean meats, poultry, fish, and low-fat dairy, or plant proteins, including legumes, nuts, seeds, and grains. Pick snacks from among these foods. They are rich in energy-boosting proteins and minerals, and are the ideal natural alternative to caffeinated and sugar-laden foods. Try peanut butter on a banana or apple, or whole-wheat crackers with a shmear of hummous, baba ganouj, some form of nut spread or butter (organic, of course), or low-fat cheese.

Fats provide a source of concentrated energy, giving your body the necessary fatty acids to accomplish many activities. Fats are also essential for carrying fat-soluble vitamins into the body, especially vitamins D, E, and K. Polyunsaturated and monounsaturated fats are the good guys. They are made from plant sources and are liquid at room temperature. Flaxseed oil and olive oil are two excellent choices. Saturated fats are the bad guys. They are generally solid at room temperature and come from meat, dairy, or tropical oil products (tropical oils include coconut and palm kernel oil). Saturated fats interfere with the removal of cholesterol from the blood. Overall, fat should represent approximately 20 to 30 percent of your daily diet, with saturated fats accounting for less than 10 percent.

On the subject of fats, too many of us eliminate all fat from our diet in an effort to remain slim. Don't do this. Remember, there are good fats and bad fats. Keep the good. They help the body produce hormones, and without proper hormone levels, we age more rapidly. Excessive fat reduction also wreaks havoc with our hair, skin, and nails. When deficient in healthy fats, the body naturally opts to use what little resources it has to nourish vital organs and sends the leftovers (if there are any!) to sustain hair, skin, and nails. In other words, the body's built-in system of checks and balances will conserve resources to save your kidneys rather than your hair. Taking in enough beans, nuts, and seeds, as well as supplementing with flax seed, borage, black currant, or evening primrose oils will provide enough essential fatty acids to serve every part of your body. By the way, eating the right amount of good fat is especially important if you do not eat meat or dairy products.

Taking the Waters

After oxygen, water is the second most important substance necessary to sustain life, and it is the most abundant substance in the body. This vital liquid accounts for approximately 60 to 80 percent of the body's weight, with our blood coming in at 90% water, and our muscles at 75% water. Your body needs water to carry out virtually all its functions, including transporting nutrients throughout the body and removing metabolic wastes (such as lactic acid) from the cells. Adequate hydration also plays a major role in regulating normal elimination, which is another vital form of detoxification.

Dehydration can cause a host of bodily malfunctions. Over long periods, insufficient water intake may accelerate aging, which is in part a drying-up process. A parched body can also cause your muscles to lose efficiency, resulting in knots and spasms. In addition, dehydration can cause irregular body temperatures, restricted joint movement, and a shutdown of several body organs.

It's unnecessary to suffer any of these ailments, since water is readily available. Make sure you get the minimum requirement of eight 8-ounce glasses every day, or optimally one quart for every 50 pounds of body weight. It's also highly recommended that we drink purified or filtered water. Try your best to reduce or eliminate ice-cold water, as this can squelch the digestive fire that optimizes metabolism of food. Furthermore, excessively cold drinks can numb the taste buds, making them less discriminating about what is being eaten and lessening our overall enjoyment of food. Remember, we're talking about our sense of taste here. Part of life's enjoyment is to revel in the taste of our foods.

The argument for bottled spring, purified, or filtered water over tap water is based on the fact that many of our faucets feed us contaminated water—water containing trace elements of pesticides, toxic chemicals, parasites, fecal matter, lead, and other toxic metals. One in five of us is drinking contaminated water. According to the Centers for Disease Control (CDC), nearly one million people get sick each year from tap water. "The problem lies in the rivers, streams, and lakes where we get our tap water. Water suppliers treat the water, but often can't get all the toxins out," warns Jane Houlihan, a senior analyst at the Washington D.C.–based Environmental Working Group (EWG). What's more, some consider the chlorine used to treat our water to be a toxin in and of itself. The Environmental Defense Fund lists chlorine as a suspected toxin for blood, liver, kidneys, nerve tissue, respiration, and skin.

If you can swing it financially, a good solution is a filter, for showers as well as sinks. These devices help decrease exposure to chlorine, pesticides, bacteria, and lead.

If the salon where you work does not have purified or filtered water, bring a supply from home in a large glass jar. Consider adding orange, lemon, and/or lime slices. Sip from this fountain of youth and health throughout the day. Also consider bringing to work a thermos of hot water, maybe with a little freshly grated ginger added to taste. This natural anti-inflammatory is detoxifying as well as a great aid for your body's digestion, absorption, and elimination processes. Try not to drink too much of any liquid with meals. It squelches the digestive process by diluting hydrochloric acid and pancreatic digestive enzymes. And remember, try to eliminate—or at least reduce—ice-cold drinks.

Sometimes, when we first begin paying attention to our water intake, it is amazing how little we actually consume. Make yourself accountable, until water consumption becomes a glorious habit. Note every sip you take during the course of a day, and continue this exercise for one week. At the end of each day, add up the ounces. Do you come up with a total of 64 ounces, or better still, one quart for every 50 pounds of body weight? You will simply not believe how great this make you feel. You will definitely want to make it a lifelong habit.

Monday

Tuesday

Wednesday

Thursday

Friday

Saturday

Sunday

Balance Your Meals

While I do not recommend taking any diet formula to extremes, I do support the basic and very popular Zone principle. My doctor introduced me to this formula, and I find that it works very well with my personal mindbody physiology. The Zone principle equates to a daily diet of 40 percent carbohydrates, 30 percent proteins, and 30 percent fat. I do not recommend eating items from any one of the food groups in excessive amounts, especially carbohydrates by themselves. For example, when enjoying a meal largely made from vegetables or fruits, you will also want a protein and a fat. This mindful adjustment will help keep your blood chemistry balanced. Also, a diet high in sugar, grains, or soda and fruit juices will severely disrupt your insulin levels. As always, listen to your body. If ever in doubt, consult your primary care physician or a nutritionist.

Guidelines for a Healthy Diet

I think many people are on overload—trying to digest too much information about what they should or should not eat. Studies are released every day, and in some cases, yesterday's research contradicts today's report. No wonder so many people simply throw their hands in the air and give up. Just remember that beyond acquiring a basic level of knowledge about food and how integral it is to your health, you also need to reach for the cleanest foods possible to feel great. Ultimately you'll want to listen to your own innate wisdom. Commit to this inner advice. And this does not mean depriving yourself of life's goodies. Yes, you can have a cookie. Yes, you can have a glass of wine. Yes, you can have fresh-baked bread and the occasional steak. Just make sure that these special treats are eaten in moderation, and make sure they're organic.

Okay, with all that said, let's get down to the specifics. We'll begin by taking a look at the U.S. government's dietary guidelines. I think these recommendations are general enough for everyone to follow.

- Eat a wide variety of foods to optimize nutrients.
- Maintain a healthy weight.
- Choose a diet low in fat, particularly saturated fat, and cholesterol.
- Choose a diet with plenty of vegetables, fruits, and whole grains.
- Use sugars only in moderation.
- Use salt and sodium only in moderation.
- If you drink alcoholic beverages, do so in moderation.

Now, these guidelines seem to make good sense, wouldn't you agree? I would, however, like to add a few footnotes. When it comes to eating a variety of foods to optimize nutrients, I urge you to begin by broadening your definition of variety. This means eating foods you've never tried before, and I bet there are plenty for you to choose from! Did you know that there are 50,000 edible plants in this world, and we eat only about 150 of them as part of our standard diet? Twenty of these plants account for about 90 percent of our food. Three of them—rice, corn, and wheat—make up half of our diet. When I say variety, I mean really push your horizons. Have you ever been to an Indian, Thai, Ethiopian, Greek, or Moroccan restaurant? Have you ever ordered the rice taffel at an Indonesian restaurant? These cultures really know how to eat a wide and diverse selection of foods.

As for these foods you are familiar with, try consuming them in different forms. Personally, I enjoy juicing my breakfast every morning—at

> **Supermarkets are all right, but it's much more fun to shop for food in nature.**
>
> *Euell Gibbons*

least one to two pounds of organic vegetables and sometimes a small amount of fruit added in for good measure. I'll add a bit of essential fatty acids (the good fats) via flaxseed oil, and sometimes unsweetened coconut for extra flavor. I change the vegetable selections every day. Juicing allows one to assimilate the maximum amount of nutrients from the veggies and fruit taken in, so drinking this morning potion provides a vitamin-packed way to start the day as well as an amazing energy high. And although it includes foods I'm already familiar with, I've modified their taste by varying my combinations, I've altered their texture, and I've even changed their appearance! When it comes to juices, be cautious about going to the local health or juice bar and ordering juices filled with simple sugars, high-fructose corn syrups, and various nonorganic ingredients.

As for the USDA's suggestion to use sugars only in moderation, I suggest that you use even less than that. Refined sugar is a detriment to your health. It weakens your immune system, depletes your life-force energy, and promotes yeast overgrowth. This last problem can snowball into even more ills. Be careful as well with your consumption of commercial low-fat foods. These devilish delights often contain high levels of refined carbohydrates, which translate into excessive sugars.

With Five You Get Twenty

Today more than ever, the subject of nutrition is very complex. This is in part due to the fact that new developments are taking place every day—particularly in the study of nutraceuticals and phytonutrients. These areas focus on how foods may be used in medicinal ways to affect our health. Many excellent books are available on this subject. Check out the resource section at the back of this book for a few suggestions.

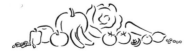

For example, when the USDA suggests that we choose a diet with plenty of vegetables, fruits, and whole grains, there's more to this statement than you might think. Several research studies suggest that five servings of fruits and vegetables a day may prevent well over 20 percent of all cancers, including colon, stomach, lung, esophagus, breast, bladder, pancreas, and prostate. The reason? Many fruits and vegetables contain powerful cancer fighters called antioxidants, and these antioxidants stabilize free radicals and halt cellular damage. The most powerful antioxidants, found in abundance in organically grown plants, include the vitamins beta carotene, C, E, and the B complex, and selenium. And for the record, organic foods have a higher vitamin, mineral, and protein content than their conventionally grown counterparts.

Some examples:

- *Cabbage*—Eaten raw or cooked, this vegetable offers high levels of antioxidants and cancer preventative constituents.
- *Carrots and sweet potatoes*—High levels of beta carotene may block the formation of tumors.
- *Chili peppers*—The capsaicin in chili peppers can reduce risk of colon, gastric, and rectal cancers while also serving to strengthen the heart and alleviate sinus conditions and chronic bronchitis. The jalapeno can protect against heart disease.
- *Citrus fruits*—These tasty treats enhance the body's detoxification systems, while the abundant vitamin C in citrus fruits and strawberries raises the activity of natural killer cells that hunt out roaming cancer cells.
- *Cranberries or cranberry juice*—Drink this sweet nectar to keep the urinary tract healthy.
- *Cruciferous vegetables*—Rich in Indole-3-carbinol, these vegetables increase the body's ability to metabolize estrogen into nontoxic form. These vegetables include, but are not limited to, broccoli, cauliflower, and cabbage.
- *Grains, seeds, and garlic*—The selenium in these items can kill cancer cells.
- *Leafy greens and nuts*—High vitamin E content may protect against genetic defects that increase cancer risk.
- *Legumes*—In particular, lentils and black beans provide significant protein and fiber, vitamins, and phytochemicals.
- *Mushrooms (maitake and shittake)*—These mushrooms both offer a valuable way to stimulate immune function.
- *Olive oil*—One tablespoon a day may counteract the cholesterol of two eggs.

- *Onions and garlic*—Organosulphur compounds in garlic protect against cancer, lower cholesterol, and help fight high blood pressure along with heart disease. Onions lower cholesterol and are helpful in controlling diabetes.
- *Parsley*—This is a valuable detoxifier for the liver.
- *Teas, green and black*—The catechin in these teas helps boost immunity, decrease cholesterol production, and reduce the risk of gastric cancer.
- *Tomatoes*—Lycopenes in this fruit (yes, the tomato is a fruit) lower your risk of cancer and lower blood pressure. Lycopene is a phytochemical (also found in red grapefruit) that is twice as powerful as beta carotene at eliminating free radicals.
- *Turmeric*—Used in curry powder, this herb is packed with antioxidants, may prevent DNA damage, and blocks tumor growth.
- *Whole grains*—A valuable source of fiber, phytochemicals, and antioxidants, fiber reduces cholesterol levels. You can get fiber in whole grains, fruits, and vegetables.

This is only the short—*very* short—list of healthy and flavorful food choices. Scientists have identified thousands of disease-fighting compounds—phytochemicals—in our food thus far . . . and research continues. Bring this into your awareness and understand that eating whole, fresh, organic foods is one of the most important preventative steps you can take toward vibrant health. Consider it health insurance.

New Cholesterol Guidelines

As for the government's recommendation that we choose a diet low in saturated fat and cholesterol, some of the most interesting recent research concerns cholesterol. Several studies report that many people don't know how to plan a cholesterol-friendly diet. Dr. Stephen Devries, a heart disease specialist at the University of Illinois at Chicago Heart Center, offers this advice. Foods labeled "cholesterol-free" might still be dangerous if they're jam packed with saturated fat, a key ingredient in hardening of the arteries. Read the label closely and make sure that there's under 2 grams of saturated fat per portion (and eat the recommended portion!). Please remember that not all fat is bad fat. The important thing is to reduce your intake of the dangerous saturated fats and trans fatty acids, the ones often found in bakery, convenience, and snack foods.

Next time you go to the grocer's, resolve to bring one or two new tastes home with you. Perhaps you could experiment with new greens like kale, mustard, and beet greens, endive, escarole, or chard. Try a variety of veggies other than the usual—kohlrabi, sun choke, yam, or Chinese cabbage. Dabble in root vegetables like turnip or parsnip. Try different grains, steel-cut or whole wheat: quinoa, amaranth, barley, kamut, or spelt. Try wild rice or basmati rice. Try tahini (sesame butter) and almond or hemp butters as an alternative to the usual peanut butter. Check out the spice aisle and add a new one, like perhaps lemongrass, cardamom, turmeric, ginseng, cilantro, sage, or curry. Purchase fruits you've never tried before, perhaps kiwi, mango, papaya, star or ugli fruit. Look for new cheeses like goat, feta, gouda, Camembert. Try edible flowers. I also urge you to become familiar with locally and regionally produced foods, and incorporate these into your diet as much as you can. Go on, be adventurous. Explore! There are so many palate-stretching foods out there.

Do some reading, investigate herb and spice sites on the Web, ask friends for recommendations, and then write down at least five unfamiliar edibles that you will purchase on your next grocery store visit.

_____

_____

_____

_____

_____

_____

Exploring the Great Pyramids

When it comes to basic nutritional recommendations, the USDA dietary guidelines that we discussed earlier are fair enough. Lately, however, there has been some disagreement over the agency's corresponding Food Guide Pyramid—the classic triangle illustrating food groups to be eaten each day. Several top-level researchers and many nutrition experts feel the USDA pyramid falls shy of perfection.

The USDA food pyramid comes from the United States Department of Agriculture, the agency responsible for promoting American agriculture—thus it is susceptible to lobbying efforts from the dairy, meat, and sugar industries. Critics claim the Department of Agriculture is incapable of remaining unbiased. Instead, many suggest that balanced, unbiased dietary recommendations should come from agencies created solely to promote and monitor health, like the Department of Health and Human Services or the National Institutes of Health.

Walter Willet, M.D., a world-renowned researcher, chairman of the Department of Nutrition at the Harvard School of Public Health, and a professor of medicine at the Harvard Medical School, took a contemporary leap forward from the USDA food pyramid and has developed the Healthy Eating Pyramid. Together with his colleagues, Dr. Willet created this dietary outline independently of any one group, basing it on global research. I encourage everyone to read Dr. Willet's book *Eat, Drink, and Be Healthy* (Simon & Schuster).

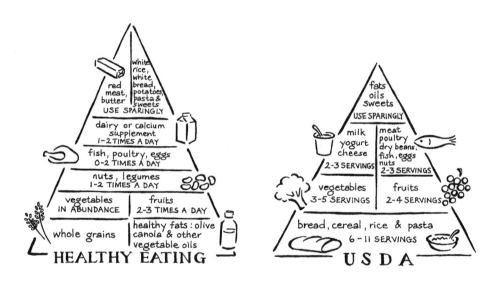

As we explore the Healthy Eating Pyramid, comparisons will be made to the USDA pyramid where applicable. You be the judge. In the meantime, I would like to suggest that you check out a few other pyramids.

There are a variety of alternative pyramids that many people don't know about. The nonprofit organization Oldways Preservation and Exchange Trust offers these alternatives at their website: www.oldwayspt.org.

Generally, these alternatives are qualitative rather than quantitative. They show you types of foods to include in your diet, and some reflect healthful eating habits from cultures around the world. In addition to the traditional USDA food pyramid, this site also includes pyramids based on Asian, Mediterranean, Latin American, and vegetarian diets. Some pyramids emphasize seafood, while others promote fresh produce. Still others are created to accommodate particular health conditions. Whatever pyramid you decide to climb depends largely on your particular nutritional goals as well as your taste buds.

Get Enough of the Good Fats

Regardless of which pyramid you choose, the Healthy Eating Pyramid sets certain parameters that I think are sensible and healthy, and they are quite simple to follow. The following pages give you a sense of these parameters.

On the subject of fats, the Healthy Eating Pyramid formula emphasizes eating less bad fat and more good, or healthy, fat. Fats from nuts, seeds, grains, fish, and liquid oils (including olive, canola, soybean, corn, sunflower, peanut, and other vegetable oils) are good for you, especially when you eat them in place of saturated and trans fats. The bad stuff includes anything with saturated or trans fats (obvious junk foods as well as red meats, whole-milk dairy, butter, and hydrogenated vegetable oils). The no-fat, low-fat message that has us believing all fat is bad is actually detrimental to our health. When we cut too far back on good fat there is a tendency to eat more carbohydrates. This generally means more highly refined or easily digested foods like sugar, white bread, white rice, and potatoes. This often leads to weight gain and potentially dangerous changes in blood fats.

It is perfectly fine to get around 30 percent of our daily calories from fats, as long as most of them are unsaturated. Read labels!

A Grain of Knowledge

Six to eleven servings of grain-based carbohydrates form the base or foundation of the USDA pyramid. The Healthy Eating Pyramid also includes grain-based carbohydrate foods but makes a distinction between refined-grain versus whole-grain carb foods. It is recommended that you eat fewer refined-grain and more whole-grain carbohydrates. Whole-grain foods are digested more slowly, are better for long-term health, and may provide some protection from diabetes, heart disease, and certain cancers and gastrointestinal problems. Highly refined carbohydrates should be used sparingly, as they are quickly digested and absorbed into the system, increasing blood sugar and insulin levels, while also raising triglyceride levels and lowering HDL (good cholesterol) levels.

Be Proactive with Protein

While the USDA pyramid advocates daily protein intake, its protein-rich edibles include a few food products that are now considered undesirable in large quantities, specifically red meats. Conversely, the Healthy Eating Pyramid includes red meat but in minimal quantities. The saturated fats in red meats, along with potentially cancer-causing compounds that form when red meat is grilled or fried, have been connected to a variety of chronic diseases. Healthy alternative protein sources include beans and nuts, as well as fish, poultry, and eggs. Animal and vegetable protein sources are separated from each other, making the animal proteins optional for those who prefer a vegetarian diet.

Eat Your Fruits and Veggies

Vegetables and fruits should have a starring role in your diet. Aside from their enormous variety of taste sensations, they also offer tremendous health benefits. You can lower your blood pressure, decrease your chances of having heart disease or a stroke, receive protection against a variety of cancers as well as gastrointestinal problems, and reduce the severity of age-related problems such as cataracts and macular degeneration. Both the USDA and Healthy Eating pyramids stress the huge importance of this food group, although the Healthy Eating option pulls potatoes into the "use sparingly" category and identifies them as a carbohydrate rather than a vegetable. Potatoes are mostly starch and are very quickly digested. This dramatically affects your levels of blood sugar and insulin.

Reaching Greater Heights

While the USDA pyramid focuses solely on food, the Healthy Eating Pyramid reaches higher, creating a comprehensive system that focuses on food groups as well as the importance of watching your weight, daily exercise, alcohol in moderation, and vitamin supplements. In my opinion, this system provides tremendous health benefits and increased longevity. How so? Let's take a closer look at the Healthy Eating Pyramid.

In Chapter Five, "Mindfulness in Motion," we covered the importance of physical activity, stressing how regular and varied activity helps keep your mindbody physiology healthy. As for watching your weight, the goal is to maintain an appropriate weight for you. This helps lessen the possibility of many debilitating diseases that can be triggered by obesity. Of course, one of several healthy ways to maintain your ideal weight is physical activity!

As for alcohol consumption, the Healthy Eating program notes recent research linking *moderate* alcohol consumption to lower rates of heart disease. It is estimated that one drink a day for women and one to two drinks a day for men can cut the chance of having a heart attack or dying from heart disease by about a third, as well as decrease the risk of ischemic stroke (caused by a clot). It is imperative, however, that you understand this: the Healthy Eating approach does not suggest that you begin drinking if you are not already doing so, and if you do use alcohol, moderation is imperative. A little bit can be beneficial; a lot is deadly.

Last but not least, the Healthy Eating program recommends taking a high-quality multivitamin every day. This suggestion is not meant to replace a healthy diet, but it can shore up nutritional inadequacies.

Use It or Lose It

Everything we've talked about in this chapter applies to society as a whole, but sometimes I feel good nutrition has particular relevance when it comes to the beauty professional. Beauty pros are especially challenged in getting optimal nourishment due to the nature of a typical workday—head-to-head bookings, standing for ten hours straight, dealing with so many different personalities. In other words, it's difficult for many of us to find time for proper nourishment, yet it's doubly important for us. And just knowing nutritional facts won't help you . . . you have to use the information wisely.

More and more salons and spas are making a point of building lunchtime into the workday. Virtually all medical offices do it, turning phones over to an answering service for a designated period of time and offering staff members a comfortable place to eat, relax, and digest. For those of you who may not yet enjoy the benefits of such policies but want to develop better eating habits, I offer the following suggestions.

Breakfast
- Make time for a nourishing breakfast every day! This helps your mindbody physiology perform at optimal level.

- Consider juicing your breakfast, mixing in some form of protein, carbohydrate, and fat. Try different combinations of whole-grain cereal, milk, peanut butter, eggs, and yogurt along with your fruits and vegetables.
- Reduce your breakfast intake of refined white flour products and limit the amount of fruit juice that you drink, including 100-percent fruit as well as organic juices.
- If you must have coffee, make it one cup and make it organic. Remember, coffee as well as alcoholic beverages can be dehydrating to your system. Minimally, drink one 8-ounce glass of water for each serving of coffee or liquor; two glasses is even better.

Lunch and Daytime Snacks
- Make thoughtful food choices during the day. If it is truly impossible to squeeze in a normal lunchtime, consider preparing petite portions of healthy nibbles that can be eaten on the run.
- Prepare an extra portion when cooking dinner. This gives you a perfect lunch for tomorrow! Many of us have more quality time to think through dinner preparation, so make an extra serving to brown bag the next day.
- Cut up veggies and add a little organic dip. Bring your healthy crudités to work the next day, and snack to your heart's content.
- Change your daily veggie and fruit choices. An apple a day is a great idea, but two apples a day won't bestow as many benefits as one apple and, say, a banana, peach, or nectarine. Think diversity!
- Invest in a wide-mouthed thermos to bring soups, chili, or casseroles to work.
- If you're a traditionalist and lunch means sandwich time, switch to whole-grain bread with grilled veggies, chicken, turkey, egg, and salmon or tuna salad, with all lunchmeats organic and nitrate free. Put delectable homemade dressings on your sandwich. Don't forget to add your veggie servings to the sandwich as well. Use romaine, spinach, or perhaps red leaf lettuce along with sliced tomatoes. Be creative. Yum!
- Bring this extra-healthy sandwich for intermittent breaktimes, cutting the sandwich into quarters and eating one energizing square between clients.
- NEVER, NEVER, NEVER skip lunch altogether or cram down a large meal in only a little time. Going a full day with spotty or no nutritional intake is detrimental over time. Taking in too much food too quickly means you'll return to work feeling tired and bloated.

Choose a Pyramid That's Right for You

What I've tried to do here is whet your appetite for good nutrition. Now go out and find the right nutritional sustenance for you. Eat mindfully and understand what your food choices are doing for you and to you. It is never too late to change bad habits and begin treating yourself to wholesome, nutritious food. Know that a healthy diet not only does beautiful things to your body's inside (think immune system and energy level) but also for your outer beauty (think hair, skin, and nails) as well as your attitude (think optimistic, resilient, and compassionate). You will function at your highest level and set the best possible example for your clients.

Nourishment Worth Sharing

Just as food nourishes your body, it also nourishes the soul. I refer not to the vitamins within food, but rather the way in which we eat—together, in groups comprised of friends, family, co-workers, even entire villages. We humans tend to build much of our social life around eating, making the experience a truly blessed and joyful happening. Think about it. You join a pal at a favorite restaurant, gather around the kitchen table with family, discuss the day as you sup with your significant other—they're all scenarios that result in nurturing the body as well as our connection with other people.

Here's a happy fact: when you eat in joyous harmony with others and in pleasant surroundings, you boost your ability to properly digest and metabolize food. This is a doubly important piece of information when you consider that so many of us have lost our mindful awareness and joy in eating. Hurry up! Fast food! Eat on the run! There is actually in existence an international movement called the Slow Food Movement. This group celebrates the joy of eating! They urge followers to recapture the celebration and ritual of dining, relishing every bite, every morsel.

For a new idea, it's really quite old, especially when you consider our ancestors' attitude toward mealtime. This was almost sacred time, when the entire family came together. Breakfast, lunch, and dinner were carefully and lovingly prepared from scratch, with ample amounts of vegetables, grains, and legumes, all delightfully seasoned with fresh herbs and spices.

As you learn to approach eating with a higher consciousness and greater awareness, I trust you will also rediscover the value of slowly, thoughtfully, and deliciously sharing mealtime with treasured people. You will come to know what your great-great-grandmother knew: the nature of your food, your appreciation for its sustenance, and the pleasure that you derive from it all meld to make the eating experience one of exquisite fulfillment.

> "Food that is eaten is divided threefold. The gross part becomes waste. The middle part becomes flesh, The subtle part becomes the mind."
>
> *Chandogya Upanishad*

Pass the Happiness, Not the Salt

Dining out with friends or family is indeed a wonderful part of our social lives, but often the people sharing your table are more beneficial to your health than the food on your plate. Restaurant food generally arrives in unnecessarily huge proportions, it tends to be packed with unhealthy ingredients, and it may be downright spoiled. To help beef up the health benefits of restaurant food, request that the chef hold off on the MSG, especially when ordering in Chinese establishments. Instead of ordering fruit juice or soda, both of which can jeopardize calcium levels in your system, request purified or filtered water, or organic herbal tea. Always try to include a salad, with dressing on the side. Avoid deep-fried food. Ask if any items on the menu come from local or regional distributors or growers, since food that has traveled a long way to reach the restaurant may be suspect. Question how things are prepared, and don't be afraid to request that your food be prepared in the most healthful way for you. All these special requests result in healthful eating choices, and while you may drive your waiter crazy, you will definitely feel better.

Now for the Eating Meditation Itself

Food has long been used as a representation of our spirituality. Overtly, this means specific foods served at religious ceremonies or traditional celebrations. A little less obvious but just as important, food also helps you express your spirituality by reflecting your personality, your passion, your mindbody physiology. Remember, we're talking about the weaving together, the union, of your mind, body, and spirit. This is what wholeness is, and when realized, it is wonderful. It becomes much easier to make healthy food selections, eat reasonable portions, and truly enjoy eating as opposed to simply filling your tummy.

It's not just the actual food on our plates that's tied to our spirituality, but also the way we digest this sustenance. To fully understand what

I mean, you should first rethink your definition of digestion. Please consider it more than the process by which we convert food into simpler chemical compounds to be assimilated by the body. I wish, instead, that you could learn to broaden this word's meaning to include not only the food we eat but also the attitude we have as we eat it.

We digest, metabolize, and assimilate all of life's experiences into who we are—into our mindbody physiology. Eating is one of these experiences, and it should be one of life's greatest pleasures. Eat with awareness of and appreciation for the nourishment you take in. I fully believe that this attitude increases your ability to assimilate nutrients. After all, we know the opposite is true: eat while you are stressed out or rushed, and your digestive system functions much less efficiently. Think heartburn, bloating, and general malaise after a particularly heavy, unhealthy meal! So it makes perfect sense to say that good digestion begins in the mind.

To learn the fine art of eating with spirit, here's how I suggest you take your next meal:

- Settle yourself into a comfortable place with your food—a place where you will not be distracted. Give your full mindfulness to the eating of this food, be it a meal or snack.
- Give thanks for every person and circumstance that went into bringing this food to you—the farmer who lovingly nurtured the soil and planted the seeds, the sun's life-giving warmth and energy that helped grow the food, all those who helped harvest the food, process it, and transport it to your grocer. Don't forget to give thanks for whoever lovingly prepared the food, including yourself if you prepared it!
- Now look closely at the food. Become intimate with its shape, form, and texture. Use all your senses. Take in the colors. Touch the food if possible. Smell the aromas. Let the food rest for a moment on your lips. Can you feel the saliva already starting to flow in your mouth? You should! All these sensory steps enact the digestive process.
- After putting the food into your mouth—not too much of it— chew thoroughly, tasting the explosion of flavors. Exercise all 10,000 taste buds.
- When it is thoroughly chewed, mentally follow the food down your esophagus and on into the stomach. Pay attention to any stomach sensations. Stay connected to this mindfulness throughout your meal.
- Do not gulp beverages during this eating meditation.

- As you continue relishing each bite, you will begin to feel the sensation of fullness.
- After finishing your meal, sit for a few moments. Breath smoothly and naturally. Give thanks again for this food and for its life-giving sustenance.
- After a few reflective moments, get up and go for a brief walk— 5 to 10 minutes will do. This will enhance the digestive process.

Now think back over the entire process. Did you feel as if you were in super-duper slow motion? That's great! This is how we were meant to take in nourishment.

The next time you eat, make it an eating meditation. Begin your meditation well before the actual act of chewing. Think about shopping for the things you truly want to eat. Once at the farmers' market, food co-op, whole foods store, or local grocery store, mindfully select these foods. Study every product label. Don't let this wonderful experience become a grab-and-run mission.

What are some ways you might make the shopping, cooking, and eating experience more thoughtful? Do you need new cookbooks? Do you need an herb and spice book that details taste sensations and possible uses? Do you need a new non-stick sauté pan so you can use less saturated fat when cooking? You might even write down a few tabletop accessories, to make your eating experience more beautiful. Think natural candles, a flower vase, pretty napkins . . . whatever!

_____

_____

_____

_____

_____

_____

_____

Prepare for Ecstasy

In addition to a spiritual connection with eating, you also want to have this mystical level of higher consciousness in food preparation. When preparing a meal or snack, you want every morsel to be prepared with love and compassion. I know that when my beloved husband James cooks our meals (he's a trained chef—I know, I know, I'm a very fortunate woman!), it is done with the very best energy possible. This is food filled with love and compassion, not only love for what's being prepared and where it came from, but also love for the process of feeding ourselves with wholesome organic food. As my husband chops, dices, mixes, marinates, spices, herbs, sauces, bakes, and steams, he is in a state of flow. And we then, with great anticipation and thankfulness, sit down to this food feast, filled with enjoyment. This has to be one of the most blissful and gratifying experiences that we would want to have in our lives. When you learn to cook with care and reverence, you, too, will discover that food, body, and nature are the same entity. The flesh of our body is the same as the flesh of our food—living breathing tissue. The energy and intelligence from our food becomes the energy and intelligence of our mindbody physiology. With each bite of food, you become one with the universe—the Earth, the water, the air, the light.

Nutrition the Ayurvedic Way

Ayurveda offers perhaps my favorite connection with nutrition as well as spirituality—a spiritual formula for nutrition. These guidelines share some elements of the USDA pyramid as well as the Healthy Eating Pyramid, but they go a step farther. This time-honored science states that a balanced meal results from the right combination of foods, but adds that for optimal nutrition, one must also consider the taste, temperature, and texture of food.

There are six specific tastes recognized: sweet, sour, salty, pungent, bitter, and astringent. The right proportion of all six tastes at each meal should eliminate food cravings—cravings that can lead to overeating and needless snacking. How do you know how to select and combine these tastes in the right proportions for you? It relates to the Ayurvedic energies or principles: air, fire, and earth. In other words, an air type, typically dry, cold, and light, can bring a balancing change to the physiology by minimizing intake of dry, cool, and light foods. These foods typically fall into the pungent, bitter, and astringent taste categories. The air type should instead lean toward sweet, sour, and salty foods. These taste categories tend to bring air types down to earth, build tissues, calm the spirit, and enhance the digestion and elimination processes. It's that simple . . . and logical.

Let's look at the six tastes and their effect on our mindbody physiology:

The Sweet Taste

The sweet taste is composed of earth and water. It encompasses the sugars and starches, which come primarily from complex carbohydrates, fats, and proteins. Sweet tastes tend to be cooling, with oily and heavy qualities. The sweet taste is very nutritive and rejuvenating, promoting regeneration of body tissues. In excess, the sweet taste may cause some disorders such as obesity, diabetes, and lethargy. Examples of sweet foods include sugar, fruit juices, honey, rice, whole-wheat bread, whole grains, pasta, milk, cream, butter, ghee (clarified butter), oils, meats, most nuts, sweet fruits (apricots, figs, dates, peaches, melons, pears, coconut), and starchy vegetables (beets, cucumbers, potatoes). This taste increases the earth energy while decreasing air and fire.

The Sour Taste

The sour taste is composed of earth and fire, and it involves fermented or acidic tastes. The sour taste's energy is hot, tends to be oily and light in nature, and stimulates the appetite while enhancing digestion. It also promotes metabolism and circulation. When enjoyed in excess, sour tastes may create such disorders as toxic build-up in the blood, excessive thirst, edema, ulcerations, and heartburn. Examples of sour taste include yogurt, cheeses, citrus fruits, green grapes, tomatoes, vinegar, salad dressings, fermented foods, and pickles. This taste increases fire and earth energy while decreasing air.

The Salty Taste

The salty taste is composed of water and fire and comes from mineral salts. Its energy heats the system, and it has oily and heavy qualities. It serves to promote better digestion, increase the appetite, mildly sedate, and aid regular elimination. As a demulcent, salty tastes help soften body tissues. Too much of this taste may cause premature graying and hair loss or thinning as well as skin diseases, blood disorders, ulcers, rashes, hypertension, and overheating. Examples of the salty taste include sea salt, rock salt, salted nuts, salted fish and meats, seafood, seaweed, and kelp. This taste increases the fire and earth energy while decreasing air.

The Pungent Taste

The pungent taste is composed of fire and air and is spicy or acrid, primarily coming from aromatic essential oils. The pungent taste's energy is heating, as well as being dry and light in nature. This taste is quite stimulating to the entire physiology, and it promotes digestion while increasing the appetite. Pungency induces sweating while clearing excess mucous or phlegm from the system. Disorders caused by excess pungency might include increased body temperature and sweating, dizziness, gastric or intestinal upset, or burning sensations in the throat, stomach, and heart. The pungent taste includes all hot peppers (chilis, cayenne, and black pepper), ginger, onion, garlic, radishes, mustard, and cloves. This taste increases the air and fire energy while decreasing earth.

The Bitter Taste

The bitter taste is composed of air and space, and it is found in alkaloids and glycosides. Its energy is cooling, and it tends to be dry and light in nature. Bitter tastes are anti-inflammatory, anti-bacterial, and detoxifying. These tastes, in small amounts, may stimulate digestion. Bitter tastes also have a reducing, depleting, and sedating effect. They also produce a drying effect on the mucous membranes, and this dryness may become excessive if too many bitter tastes are taken. Other disorders may include emaciation, fatigue, and dizziness. Examples include bitter greens, rhubarb, turmeric, sprouts, fenugreek, tonic water, and alkaloids (caffeine and nicotine). This taste increases the air energy while decreasing fire and earth.

The Astringent Taste

The astringent taste, which is composed of earth and air, comes from tannins. There is a puckering effect from many of these foods. The energy of this taste is cooling and dry, and the taste has a drying, firming, and compacting effect on the physiology. If astringent tastes are taken in excess, some disorders may include excessive dryness, constipation, retention of gas, obstruction of circulation, and heart pain. Examples include unripe bananas, apples, cranberries, pomegranates, broccoli, cabbage, cauliflower, lettuce, spinach, beans, lentils, and tea. The astringent taste increases the air energy while decreasing fire and earth.

To Review

In relating the six Ayurvedic tastes to different mindbody constitutions, here's a general guideline.

Air

Favor: oily, warm, and heavy foods from the sweet, sour, and salty tastes.

Limit intake of: pungent, bitter, or astringent tastes as well as cold foods and cold or iced drinks, light or raw foods.

Fire

Favor: cool or moderately warm foods from the sweet, bitter, and astringent tastes.

Limit intake of: sour, salty, and pungent tastes, as well as hot foods and drink.

Earth

Favor: light, dry, and warm foods from the pungent, bitter, and astringent tastes.

Limit intake of: sweet, sour, and salty taste, cold food and drinks as well as rich desserts.

You may wonder how to balance these tastes in your meal, whether you are feeding an entire family or just yourself. Proportionately, you want to eat more of the vegetables and salads if you are an earth type—not omitting the bread, rice, or pasta, just eating smaller portions of these sweet tastes. If eating any animal foods, take in small, measured quantities. It is the reverse for air types. Help yourself to more of the sweet tastes (in the form of fruits and vegetables, as well as starches and proteins—grains, pastas, rices, meats) and less of the raw or cold salads and vegetables. In other words, it's not about abstaining or gorging on various tastes. Rather, enjoy them all but in proportions that reflect your mindbody type. You always want to get at least a bit of all six tastes at every meal. This helps prevent cravings even when you are not truly hungry.

It is important to understand that this information should serve only as a general guide to optimizing nutrition for your mindbody constitution. I do not suggest you become obsessive, because this in and of itself can cause needless stress and anxiety. After all, an Ayurvedic diet is designed to nourish the body and restore balance.

Serve Yourself More Than Food

The final area of nutrition I feel compelled to address is actually anti-nutrition, or more clearly put, the negative results when we consume food in order to fill an emotional need. We all need to be very careful to never, ever confuse emotional and spiritual hunger with physical hunger.

Occasionally, we all walk this calorie-strewn path. Did you have an unusually lousy day? A cheesecake, eaten out of the container with a spoon, erases tension for some. Did your date stand you up? A pint of ice cream should chill the blues. Did a client specifically request blonde streaks but decide after you were done that red really would have been better? This calls for fries with lots of gooey fake cheese on top! It's when we constantly eat unhealthy foods, hoping to solve deeply rooted emotional problems, that serious trouble arises. When this happens, you can bet a donut that you'll have even greater emotional issues as well as suffering from serious physical health problems.

If distressed over a traumatic, life-altering experience, I urge you to do three things. First and foremost, consult a specialist. This person can be a qualified therapist or psychiatrist, a religious leader, or your primary care physician. At the very least, one of these persons will be able to lead you to the right expert for your particular issue.

Secondly, I suggest you speak with a nutrition expert. You may be so immersed in your food obsession and misplaced need to constantly feed yourself that you can no longer comprehend a healthy diet. A nutrition specialist will put you back on track and help you create a healthy eating plan. Once you begin to notice changes in your physical as well as emotional well-being, you should be able to go solo.

My third recommendation is that you introduce yourself to meditation and prayer. For many, these are vital keys to turning food compulsions around. The repetitive quality of both meditation and prayer will help you to slow down, clear your mind of clutter, and thus put you in a better position to clearly see reality. As you become enveloped in reality, you should find food falling into its proper place, freeing you to advance on the path toward healthy emotional fulfillment. Now you should find that you are free to fill yourself up with relationships, creative outlets, or whatever it is you've been craving— and trying so obsessively to replace with food.

The next time you take a lunch break, visit your favorite restaurant, or prepare a meal at home, ask yourself: "Are these food choices going to make me feel good? Will they optimize my energy levels and ultimately my health and well-being?"

Eventually—with your knowledge about the fundamentals of healthy eating, and your desire for tasty, whole foods—you will reply to your own questions with a resounding YES.

Write down all the foods you ate at your last meal. If you used any boxed, canned, or bagged foods, write down the ingredients printed on the container label. (Note the megachemicals in the food if applicable!) No one's testing you here, so be honest! Underline the foods that were not serving you well. Now describe a similar meal, replacing the energy-depleting or downright unhealthy items with good alternatives. For example, if you had nachos with fake cheese, try replacing this taste desire with homemade quesadillas and homemade salsa—all organic, of course.

My last meal consisted of:

_____

_____

_____

_____

_____

_____

A similar but healthier meal alternative would be:

_____

_____

_____

_____

_____

_____

Food for Thought

Please consider the following:

- Take in as many whole, natural foods as you can, and eliminate as many processed and refined foods as possible. Highly processed or refined foods lack nutrients, and the chemical and artificial additives are toxic to our systems. Analyze the ingredient label on foods that come in a box, bag, or can. Unless the label states certified organic or minimal processing, take a pass.

- Choose USDA-certified organic grains, herbs, spices, fruits, vegetables, and animal foods whenever possible. This automatically limits your exposure to pesticides and nitrate-laden fertilizers. These chemicals disrupt proper functioning of the liver, kidneys, and endocrine/hormonal systems. A certified organic label also assures you that any meat, poultry, or dairy product you select was not treated with antibiotics or growth hormones before landing in your grocery store. If you are interested, there are plenty of great books out there that can give you 100 more reasons to reach for the USDA-certified organic label.

- Bolster your energy levels by eliminating or reducing your intake of caffeine and simple concentrated sugars. When you do imbibe, make sure your coffee, cream, and sugar are all organic. Coffee or caffeinated beverages stimulate our central nervous system, which causes the adrenal glands to release stored sugar in the liver. In addition, there is also the release of cortisol, a stress hormone, and accelerated formation of free radicals. As for the quick lift that caffeinated beverages and sugar give us, you should know that this lift is short-lived. Your system will soon cycle downward and need another caffeinated beverage or sweet. This yo-yo cycling eventually creates adrenal exhaustion, overstimulation of insulin, and physiological addiction.

- Replace caffeinated drinks with herbal alternatives. Essiac, Pau d'Arco, dandelion, and nettle are all amazing purifying and cleansing herbal concoctions. Chamomile is calming. Peppermint is invigorating. Yerba mate, with its earthy flavor, serves as a great coffee substitute. Stevia (available in small packages) and licorice steeped in a tea both serve to healthfully sweeten tea.

- Make your food choices something to smile about. The Centers for Disease Control report that one in three of us have untreated tooth decay. You should also know that gum disease has been linked to debilitating conditions such as heart disease. To protect your pearly whites, try to select only clean foods—they can reduce build-up of toxicity in your system, which in turn can limit gum and teeth problems. Floss and brush after every meal. Consider using a tongue scraper in the morning—readily available in most oral hygiene aisles, this device helps remove build-up of toxins—and visit your dentist regularly, a minimum of once a year, and twice is even better.

- Listen to your body. Witness how your body reacts to food choices. Observe how energetic you feel after eating certain foods, and conversely pay close attention to how certain foods or beverages result in a depletion of energy.

I hope this chapter motivates you to really see what it is that food does for and to our mindbody physiology. Nutritional sustenance is so much more than the physical need to eat. It is part of an amazing physical, mental, and emotional process, and when done mindfully, this process ups the power to control our beauty and wellness. Now go munch on some fresh green beans, with a drizzle of basil-spiked olive oil, and enjoy life.

Notes:

Chapter Seven

Sensory Awareness

66 Remember only the beautiful things
that you have felt, and seen, and
experienced. If your five senses behold
only the good, then your mind will be
a garden of blossoming soul qualities. 99

Paramahansa Yogananda

- *I was touched by what you said,* or *We lost touch with each other.*
- *Something smells fishy,* or *She has a nose for news.*
- *That's music to my ears,* or *Sounds good to me.*
- *I see what you mean,* or *She began to see the light.*
- *The experience left a bad taste in my mouth,* or *She has good taste.*
- *Have you lost your senses?*

The senses serve as metaphors and poetic phrases for so many of life's emotions and experiences. Truly, it is through the senses that we fully experience life's diverse and rich offerings. We have already visited many sensory experiences in *Body of Knowledge,* but there are more yet to explore. So what are we waiting for? Let's investigate.

We experience our outer world largely through our five primary senses. This amazing quintet offers a sacred entry into our consciousness. Every moment of every day, we receive impressions from stimuli through specific bodily organs—sense organs—and the nerves associated with them.

> The human body is its own best apothecary. The most successful prescriptions are those filled by the body itself.
>
> *Norman Cousins*

These impressions are transmitted as sensations to the brain, where they are then transformed into electrical energy and dispatched to the entire mindbody physiology—resulting in pleasure, pain, and a billion other experiences.

This marvelous process is the reason I like to remind people that inside the head rests a brain—one element of the mind. Truly, the *mind* doesn't dwell in the brain at all. The mind travels throughout your entire body, riding along hormones and enzymes. Every cell in your entire body has a mind. If you come from a place of balance, all these single cells experience a synergy with one another. It is as if they are all lovingly talking to and interacting with each other, and ultimately communicating with the brain.

When we have stressful or distasteful experiences, dissonance can take place in our cellular community. Certain cells may decide to become renegades, separating from the community, and potentially producing disharmony within the cellular community.

Sensory awareness, as well as modulation of our sensory impressions, can profoundly strengthen this cellular community, and thus our experiences in consciousness. We can choose experiences that are life-affirming and enriching, or we can choose toxic experiences that leave noxious sensory impressions on our mindbody physiology. It is through mindfully gazing, touching, listening, eating, and feeling that we experience and celebrate the awe-inspiring possibilities in our presence here.

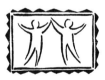 This mindfulness also extends outward into the environment, affecting how we interact with people, places, and situations. It is through the senses that we celebrate our true divinity—our alignment with spirit. This is when we connect with our truest nature.

Along our journey through this Body of Knowledge, we have explored sensory awareness as it relates to taste, or nutrition. We have also discussed at length our sixth sense—the divine sense, as I like to call it—with which we are able to see within the mind's eye and visualize our dreams as reality. This is where we commune with spirit. Now let's explore the

> **Oh**, that the water softens the rocks with time, may thy hands craft my body soft like the weathered rocks.
>
> *Anonymous*

remaining four senses—touch, smell, sight, and sound. Just like our sense of taste and our sixth sense, these, too, represent ways in which we can heighten our professional and personal experiences.

Touch Me, Feel Me— Our Sense of Touch

Touch is such a primal need, and one of our most intimate and powerful forms of communication. If you work in a salon or a spa, you know the value of touch, for it is through touch that you do your job. This is how you make human connections and ascertain information in order to make intelligent decisions. As for the person for whom you perform a beauty or wellness service, his or her senses register your touch, and the mindbody physiology will react.

How strongly does the sense of touch affect our perception of a moment? In one study, librarians were instructed to go about their business as usual, but subtly touch only some of the patrons they came in contact with. Later all the patrons were quizzed about their library experience. Those who were touched unanimously and enthusiastically gave their library experience two thumbs up—even reporting that the librarian smiled at them, when in fact the librarian did not. Those who were not touched generally had no opinion about their library experience.

In another study, it was found that restaurant servers received greater gratuities when they touched a diner, albeit very subtly on a hand or shoulder.

Yet more research into touch shows that cultures that are predisposed to showering their infants and children with appropriate, loving, and plentiful physical attention generally exhibit lower rates of adult violence. Are these cultures less violent because it is permissible for adults to caress their children, and the act of touching a child is in and of itself soothing to everyone involved? Or is it because children who receive hugs and

> **One whose physiology is in balance and whose body, mind, and senses remain full of bliss, is called a healthy person.**
>
> *Shushruta Samhita*

kisses tend to grow up into less violent adults? Actually, it's yes to both questions, and the subsequent combination of results gives these openly affectionate societies a more compassionate disposition.

Taken together, these studies point out how touch can affect our present-moment awareness as well as potentially an entire cultural personality. We absolutely must realize that touching is a form of communicating, and that the benefits go beyond physical health. If you touch others with sensitivity, you relate to them with sensitivity. This is so important for all of us to understand. After all, we are, by our calling, in constant touch with touch. It's an integral part of what we do as beauty and wellness professionals.

The Skin We're In

We experience so much through the skin we're in. Our skin, the body's largest organ, includes as many as five million touch receptors, with 3,000 in a single fingertip. These touch receptors send messages along the spinal cord to the brain. A simple touch with loving intent—a hand on a shoulder, an arm around a waist, a warm handshake, and, yes, a hug—can reduce the heart rate and lower blood pressure. Touch also stimulates the brain to produce endorphins, the body's natural pain suppressors. Maybe this is why a mother's hug can make almost anything all better.

Through our skin, we can feel tickling, repulsion, arousal, tension, heat, cold, love, and a billion more feelings—all as sensations that arise from the sensory impressions we take in through our skin and sense of touch. What we feel, and thus the expressions that these feelings produce, can even make indelible marks in our skin. (I'm thinking here about frown lines and laugh lines.)

The Professional Touch

We are, in essence, professional touchers. As we provide a beauty and wellness service, whether it's a haircut, manicure, pedicure, facial, or massage therapy session, we touch the person seated in our chair or reclining upon our massage table—physically, emotionally, and, yes, spiritually.

On a physical level, touch is a powerful healer. Our touch elicits physiological changes that can nurture and calm. It's true! Muscles relax, stress is reduced, and a calm comes over the person being touched. In addition to the sensitive, loving touch you engage in with each client from the beginning to the end of any particular service, communication with a client through touch can also include the grounding/centering ritual that I addressed in an earlier chapter, a hand and arm massage, or a neck and shoulder rub along with or after shampooing. Remember, we're talking about our right livelihood here, our calling, not just a *job*.

How deep this touching experience goes varies from client to client. In other words, time will give you a better idea of how much touch and what kind of touch most profoundly benefits each client. You will have some clients who are quite touchy-feely and want the works. Other clients will set boundaries—verbally or nonverbally—as to the amount and type of touch they prefer. As a beauty professional, it is your responsibility to know and respect these boundaries.

If you explain what it is that you're doing or going to do and why, your client will be more apt to feel at ease with your touch and more inclined to communicate what they like or don't like. It's all about our openness and artful ability to communicate—not leaving anything to the client's imagination. Even for massage therapy, a traditionally silent activity, communication remains key, although your timetable for conversation will change. You should skip conversation during the session; instead explain exactly what you will be doing before the treatment actually begins. However, invite a client to speak up during the session if any needs or requests arise. It is through gentle, free-flowing conversation that you can encourage a client to ultimately feel comfortable in requesting that any part of the treatment be adjusted—pressure, temperature, amount of oil, etc.

As a professional toucher, consider all the ways you connect physically with your clientele. I am not talking about the obvious here, but about the subtle extra touches that you do or could provide to clients, helping them relax and really sink into any particular beauty and wellness service. For instance, do you provide a scalp massage before shampooing? Do you provide a shoulder massage after a skin care treatment? An arm massage before, during, or after a manicure? Do you ruffle, move, twist, and push the hair around before beginning a cut, in order to get a visual preview of how a design will look? Hey, this last is not as direct as a massage, but it counts!

_____

_____

_____

_____

_____

Massage and the Mindbody Physiology

An integral part of touch, as it pertains to the beauty and wellness professional, is massage. Do you know what sustained touch through massage therapy can do? This is not a rhetorical question! You really should know this answer in order to best do your job. Whether you're a beauty pro in an environment where massage is offered, or you're the massage therapist, it is holistically part of your sphere of influence, and it can have a dynamic effect on you. I know well what massage therapy is capable of accomplishing. Like breathing, meditation, organic food, and plenty of physical activity, massage is an area where I simply will not compromise. I see my massage therapist every other week. She helps me feel whole. And she coaxes out those stressful holding patterns that are bound up inside my muscles. In addition to just plain making me feel good, massage relaxes me, reduces stress, improves blood circulation, increases flexibility, enhances range of motion, and raises energy levels.

How does all this happen? Well, when your skin is stroked, whether in a full-body massage or simply a neck, shoulder, scalp, or foot rubdown, a pharmacy of natural feel-good chemicals is released into your bloodstream. This includes, but is not limited to, natural growth hormones, natural anti-depressants, natural tranquilizers, natural pain relievers, immunomodulators, and vasodilators (which serve to open and dilate blood vessels). Massage can also dramatically increase lymph flow, moving toxins out of the system. This assistance with detoxification is so very important because the skin is a primary pathway for detoxification.

What else can massage do, you ask? Well, it enhances immune function and lowers levels of the stress hormones cortisol and norepinephrine. Some types of massage seem to release old injuries held in a muscle's memory, allowing the healing process to proceed. Massage can even stimulate increased production of the lubricating fluid between muscles and fascia that is critical for internal organ health. Massage also stimulates the vagus, one of twelve cranial nerves that influence a variety of bodily functions. One branch of the vagus travels to the gastrointestinal tract, where it facilitates the release of food absorption hormones like insulin and glucose, making food absorption more efficient.

All these points illustrate the incredibly rejuvenating and healing benefits that stroking or massaging the skin can have for our mindbody health. This is important information for you to personally bring into your awareness, not only so you understand the healthful benefits massage can bring to you, but also so you can share this information with your clients. Give clients the facts and then refer them to a massage therapist—either in your salon or spa or in your referral network. Also, a client armed with the facts, may be able to sink more deeply into relaxation as you provide a scalp or neck and shoulder massage before the scheduled beauty treatment.

Begin with Yourself First

The information that we've explored thus far is vital in communicating the importance of touch to your clients. First, you will want to bring this information into your consciousness. Believe it, experience it, and learn the value of massage, so that you may impart it to others. As with everything we've discussed in this book, it all begins with your own extreme self-care.

If you have not experienced the full joy of touch yourself, make an appointment for a massage therapy treatment. Today. If the salon or spa where you work does not offer massage therapy, contact the American

Massage Therapy Association for qualified recommendations. I could wax poetic about the virtues of touch until both of us are blue in the face, but until you experience its healing powers for yourself, you will never truly comprehend all I say.

A Style for Every Type

I do want to emphasize that there are many types of massage therapy, along with a variety of beneficial results. The traditional Swedish massage involves manipulation of the muscles and tissues. The Oriental healing arts concentrate on pressure points and other subtle systems in the body. This area includes Shiatsu, which focuses on pressure points and the body's energy flow. Reflexology is a foot or hand massage technique based on the centuries-old Chinese theory that areas of the feet and hands correspond directly to other body parts, namely organs, glands, and joints. Through gentle pressure and manipulation, blockages and tensions can be released. Then there are massage techniques such as acupressure, aromatherapy, Ayurvedic, cranial sacral therapy, deep tissue, Esalen, lymphatic therapies, myofascial release, Ohashiatsu, Thai-style, trigger point/myotherapy, and Watsu (water massage), to name only a few.

Many massage professionals use a combination of these techniques, adjusting them as needed to customize therapies. For example, given my muscularity, my massage therapist uses a deep neuromuscular massage on me, coupled with trigger point therapy. This is ideally suited for my needs. Another individual may want less pressure and more calming strokes, given their level of need and comfort.

As a massage therapist myself, one of the most important things I have learned is this: always be aware of the power of your hands and the energy they can transfer. To grasp this point, try closing your eyes and "listening" to the tissues and bones beneath your hands as you give a massage. Imagine the structure of the body. Envision this body with a sense of wholeness and interconnectedness—rather than seeing the body as separate parts. Intuitively performing a massage with this intent and in this manner enhances the quality of the experience for both persons involved!

There is such a variety of massage knowledge and expertise out there, it is probably wisest for me to simply ignite your interest and then urge you to seek more information on your own. The Internet can be very beneficial in this regard. Numerous courses, videos, and books are also available. In addition, I've offered several interesting references in the resource section of this book. In the meantime, I hope you now realize the tremendous healing and relaxation benefits that touch and specifically massage can bring into any person's life. They can be very blissful indeed!

Massage Massages So Many Skills

For myself and many of my fellow beauty professionals, learning massage therapy has led to making the connection between body, mind, and spirit, and studying this fine art has also allowed us to hone a few vital skills.

First there's the ability to listen, an integral part of "people skills." When giving a massage, you must be totally and intuitively tuned in to your client's comfort and ease with the experience. You need to have complete present-moment awareness in order to hear cues—verbal or nonverbal leads—that tell you that your pressure is too hard or not hard enough, that too little oil is being used and undesirable friction is being created on the skin, or too much oil is being used for a client's personal tastes. A key to successful massage therapy is communication.

Learning massage therapy also gives one a keen insight into the importance of environment, or ambiance. I've learned how to choose the proper lighting, create quiet surroundings, and work with quality products and equipment, all chosen to deliver the most delightful massage experience. Of course, part of ambiance is aroma and music, both indivisible from massage therapy and quite engaging for all the senses. After collecting all this valuable information, spread your wisdom around. Use your knowledge about creating the perfect setting to make your work station or massage therapy space more inviting. Don't forget to bring this knowledge home, using it to make your personal headquarters engaging for visitors as well as yourself!

Self-Massage

As part of giving yourself the love and attention you deserve (because you are lovable—give yourself a positive affirmation here), don't forget to give yourself a daily self-massage. It's a great way to wake up or bed down.

Begin by mixing a bit of organic plant oil with a favorite essential oil. Select your essential oil for its calming and/or cooling properties or for its stimulating benefits—whatever you need at that moment. Be sure to give yourself the gift of time, at least 5 minutes but preferably 10, so you can mindfully move through a total body rubdown. Begin with your scalp and work down to the tips of your toes. Be with the process and remember to breathe. After your massage is complete, bathe in a gentle, organic body wash.

Use self-massage wherever and whenever the yearning arises. Sore muscles or inflamed tendons? Spend a few moments massaging them. Feeling lethargic? Stimulate your get-up-and-go. Feet hurt? Kick off the shoes and spend a few minutes with your tootsies. Tummy upset? Gently massage your stomach in a clockwise motion. A little too jazzed to go to bed? Treat yourself to a scalp or foot massage, crawl into bed afterwards, and enjoy blissful sleep, not to mention moisturized skin and scalp.

By all means, don't forget your hands! Our hands as messengers of touch and emotion will greatly benefit from diligent care. To be quite blunt, it's not a pleasant experience when the beauty professional touches you with dry, cracked, chapped skin. Keep your hands conditioned by exercising and stretching them regularly. Massage regularly with certified organic hand lotions. Be gentle, and be thorough. These are your healing hands. Spend some time loving them.

As for your own personal situation, it is difficult for your skin's five million touch receptors to send messages to the brain when your skin is in poor condition. Be meticulous in caring for your own skin—all of it! Remember, your skin is your body's largest organ and reflects so many choices that you make each and every day toward beauty and wellness. A consistent holistic regimen of cleansing, toning, moisturizing, exfoliating, and protection with organic skin care products is a good beginning. When you combine it with stress management, good nutrition, physical activity, adequate hydration, and healthful lifestyle choices—like moderating sun exposure and not smoking—your skin will radiate beauty.

I am going to do some shameless self-promotion here. I penned a book called *Radiant Beauty: Your Healthy and Organic Guide to Total Body Well-Being* (Rodale Press, 2001). Please do pick up a copy. I delve into skin care in this book at great length, along with organic hair care; organic beauty care for the hands, feet, and nails; and a wide variety of approaches toward organic beauty for the senses—all ways to physically care for the wellness and attractiveness of our sensory organs as well as accentuate our sensory experiences. This book would be a perfect complement to the one you're reading right now!

I do hope that this information on touch has touched your world— and that in turn you will regard your loving touch as the holistic and healing ritual it is.

> 6 6 I remember the grass beyond the door,
> the sweet keen smell around the shore. 9 9
>
> *Dante Gabriel Rossetti*

Blissful Sleep

Adults require somewhere between 7 and 9 hours of sleep each night. A large number of us get only 6.5 hours or less. Such chronic sleep deprivation not only makes you feel tired, but it can also slow your reaction time, lower your IQ, and weaken your immune system. So, try to get the optimal amount of sleep. Take valerian tincture before bed, have a cup of chamomile tea or a cup of organic milk with a bit of honey. Luxuriate in a warm bath. Most certainly, give yourself a foot and scalp massage in order to calm down and balance your brain waves. Sweet dreams!

Heaven Scent—Our Sense of Smell

It was Heaven Sent perfume that I wore in high school. My husband, who was my boyfriend back then, wore Brut. Smelling these fragrances today brings back a flood of memories from the good old days. We all have similar stories, where memory and emotions intimately connect with aroma. Fragrances have the power to stir something deep within us—and for good reason!

A person's nose contains millions of scent receptor cells, and each of these cells has microscopic hairlike nerve endings called cilia. Every single one of these cilia has a receptor that binds with odor molecules. When aromas bind with these receptors, electrical impulses are sent to the brain's smell center. This signals the cerebral cortex to send information to the limbic system—the seat of our emotions, memories, intuition, and sexual response. The limbic system also affects hormone levels, influences the immune system, and interacts with the neocortex area of the brain. Hence the connection between our sense of smell and our thoughts, emotions, desires, and moods.

And also remember that your sense of smell enhances the digestion process, which we spoke of in

Chapter Six, "Nourishing Wisdom." To jog your memory, we talked of how smelling your food before even taking that first bite starts the digestive process by getting saliva to flow in the mouth.

In addition to spurring memories, emotions, and the digestive process, smells can potentially effect great healing—whether internal or external. We can use aroma as a form of therapy to boost confidence, help de-stress, detoxify, and nurture our bodies, soothe aching muscles, improve the skin, enhance metabolic and other bodily functions, and purify our environment. In addition, aromas can accelerate learning, quell anxiety, soothe and calm, dispel anger, stimulate and motivate, engender love, enhance sexual desire, enhance appetite, increase blood circulation, mois-turize, tone, and provide astringency for the skin, hair, and nails . . . the list goes on and on and on. It is definitively proven that aromas have real and therapeutic benefits, affecting us physically, mentally, emotionally, and spiritually. Becoming familiar with all these benefits allows us to integrate aromas intelligently into our personal and work environments.

The connection between scent and emotion runs deep. Here are a few evocative scents. Think about each one, smell it in your "mind's nose." Does the scent connect to an experience for you?

- Fresh-mown grass
- The innocent smell of baby powder
- The incense you light before meditation
- Fresh bread baking
- Cabernet Sauvignon, or any wonderful fruit of the vine
- Rosemary or basil from the garden, crushed between your fingers
- Crushed mint leaves
- Cinnamon
- Fresh vegetable soup bubbling on the stove
- Fresh-brewed coffee
- The smell of fall
- The smell of rain
- The smell of any flower
- The musky, sexually enticing pheromones we put out

Now write down any other special scents that you associate with special memories or emotions.

_____

_____

_____

_____

_____

_____

_____

_____

_____

_____

Toxic Smells

Most certainly, there are toxic as well as enticing smells in our environment. Consider your environment at home and at work, including the outdoor air quality in your neighborhood, outgassing from volatile organic compounds, chemicals from the products we use, cigarette smoke, traffic congestion, and other factors. This is where the importance of getting *fresh* air becomes paramount.

Getting fresh air does not mean simply standing in your backyard—it goes deeper than this. Pollutants strip the air of its natural healing components—specifically the negative ion. Negative ion environments are found at the ocean's edge, in pine forests, by waterfalls, and generally anywhere just after a lightning storm. Negative ion environments can simultaneously calm you and make you feel exhilarated. When negative ion environments are disrupted by pollution, the result is positive ionization, which can make you feel fatigued, depressed, tense, and irritable, along with producing possible physical effects including frequent headaches, allergies, and even difficulty breathing. Denise Linn delves deeply into this subject in her book *Sacred Space* (Ballantine, 1995).

To make certain you're getting enough *fresh* air:

- Consider purchasing an ionizer for your home and work environments.
- Make sure you can open your windows to circulate air, and that you have an efficient air-filtration system.
- Surround yourself with green plants—placing the indoor variety around you as well as placing yourself outdoors among lush foliage. This allows you to take in prana-rich air, or the breath that these plants release.

Personal Best

When it comes to our sense of smell, I would be remiss if I skipped the issue of personal hygiene—a very important matter for us beauty and wellness professionals. As a one-time salon manager, I had the dubious honor of taking employees aside and talking to them about any offensive odors—perspiration scents not kept in check, perfumes applied with a ladle rather than a spritz, or bad breath due to smoking, poor oral hygiene, or garlic-loaded lunches.

How many clients do not return to visit a beauty professional for reasons attributable to personal hygiene? This is difficult to determine, but probably more than we care to admit. Bring your own personal body scents into your consciousness, and make sure you smell fresh throughout the day. Do a regular self-smell test. This includes oral as well as body hygiene. Keep a toothbrush and dental floss at work for after-lunch attention. And if your afternoon walk makes you perspire, splash a little cool water on your face and freshen up those underarms instead of dousing yourself in perfume.

As for associates who have odious odors, there are sensitive ways to address these issues. Come from a place of genuine loving-kindness, and you will most likely be well received. Truthfully, in discussing odd personal odors, you may be providing a huge health service. Unpleasant odors emanating from someone can be connected to medical issues or a build-up of toxins in the system. This may require medical treatment and/or detox. If you or someone you care for cannot eliminate an offensive odor through traditional means (i.e. better oral or body hygiene), this person should seek out a professional health practitioner's advice.

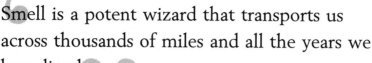

> **Smell** is a potent wizard that transports us across thousands of miles and all the years we have lived . . .

Helen Keller

Give Me the Real Deal

On the subject of perfumes and associated products, let's take a closer look. I'm sure every one of you can relate to being around someone who indeed must have bathed in his or her favorite fragrance. Often a product's overbearing aroma is exacerbated by its synthetic qualities. Synthetic coloring and synthetic fragrances are the two top ingredients in products that elicit unfavorable responses in certain individuals, and even invoke allergic reactions. These reactions may also be part of multiple chemical sensitivity disorder, in which a cumulative assault of chemicals on the mindbody physiology creates a fairly intense problem that can be life-altering.

It really is important to honor and surround ourselves with the most natural fragrances possible—including hair and skin care products, work and household cleaning products, and the candles, incense, and essential oils we use. This will dramatically decrease possible negative reactions to scent. There are even some spas with a no-fragrance policy. These spas have definitely found their niche, offering a safe haven for scent-sensitive clients.

Aromatherapy

Aromatherapy is widely practiced in Europe. Medical schools in France regularly teach students how to prescribe essential oils. Stateside, more doctors, dentists, psychologists, and nurses are beginning to use aromatherapy in medical settings, such as hospitals, hospices, and nursing homes. Why all the attention to aromatherapy? Because this truly delightful art and science based on scent can alleviate stress, calm the fight-or-flight response, promote alertness, induce sleep, and increase appetite.

If you are working in the beauty and wellness profession in any capacity, chances are you have some familiarity with—or even a proficient working knowledge of—aromatherapy. It is very important that we be able to intelligently educate our clients as to what aromatherapy is and what it is *not*.

Aromatherapy has become a catchphrase for so many products flooding our stores—from aromatherapy personal care products to aroma therapeutic accessories for the home. And while I fully applaud the attention to this healing therapy, I am concerned that many of these products contain essential oils—or should I say fragrances—that are diluted and possibly synthesized, and do not truly reflect what 100-percent-pure essential oils can accomplish. High-quality essential oils are unadulterated and have no synthetic fillers, suspenders, or added mineral oil. Read the label of any aromatherapy product you wish to purchase, looking for 100-percent-pure essential oils, preferably organic.

Personally, I enjoy using essential oils on a daily basis. I inhale them neat (inhaled straight from the bottle, on an organic cotton ball, a handkerchief, or in aromatherapy jewelry), or I may use them in a diffuser. I add them to my organic plant oil for self-massage. I have a small clay diffuser containing essential oils in my car. The essential oil I choose at any given time depends on how I feel at that moment. If I need to de-stress and calm down, I may choose calming oils like lavender or neroli. If I need to give myself an energy boost, I may opt for rosemary or lemongrass. And I certainly blend essential oils together. Many high-quality essential oils can also be purchased in blended form.

If you are not presently using essential oils in your work environment, to help ignite an interest in them, start with the following simple aromatic practices. Begin with a few favorites, then slowly expand your repertoire of essential oil usage as you become more knowledgeable. Naturally, make sure that aromatherapy is acceptable in your work environment. First, ask if your ideas are acceptable, and if you get the thumbs up, then be sure to also ask if any coworkers would like to join you in your aromatic education.

- Float a few drops of a favorite essential oil in an attractive small container at your work station.
- Light a high-quality aromatherapy candle.
- Add a drop or two of essential oil to the manicure or pedicure water.
- Add a few drops to your massage oil.
- Enhance a shampoo or conditioning service by adding a drop or two of an essential oil into the liquids used.

There are many excellent courses, CDs, videos, and books, that can help you learn about the more than 700 essential oils in existence. And certainly spend extra time studying the essential oils pertinent to your own needs, your clients' needs, and the general beauty services you provide.

Finally, there are some very specific cautions about using essential oils, and any reputable training program will include discussion of these issues. For instance, you should be aware of different applications and usage proportions with a carrier oil. There's also the importance of proper storage, the need for a patch test, incompatibility with certain medical conditions and medications, or restricted usage for anyone who is pregnant—all very important information to learn before you begin using pure essential oils.

I believe we have sufficiently explored how our sense of smell and the world of scents can dramatically affect us through our memories, our emotions, and, most certainly, our physicality. My goal here has been to expand your awareness about the value of our olfactory sense—and perhaps inspire you to take this awareness to a new level in your own experiences. Our sense of smell can bring us great pleasure and healing. Bring this as wholly into your consciousness as you can, for your own pleasure and for the pleasure and healing that you can provide to clients.

Making Sense of the Scents

Aromatherapy is defined as the art and science of using essential oils (the volatile oils distilled from plants) to relax, balance, and stimulate the body, mind, and spirit. These aromatic concentrates are generally steam-distilled from a variety of flowers, roots, leaves, barks, and resins, or cold-pressed from the rinds of citrus fruits. Every essential oil has its own distinct odor, stimulating an array of emotional, psychological, and physical responses. Oils are massaged into the skin in diluted form, inhaled, or placed in baths. Essential oils work by releasing a gaseous vapor into the air. When inhaled, the vaporized molecules are absorbed into the bloodstream through the olfactory receptors in the nostrils and through the lungs. When applied externally through bath, hydrotherapy, or massage, essential oils not only work their wonders on the multiple layers of the skin but are also absorbed through the skin and carried by the bloodstream to muscle tissues, joints, and organs. Aromatherapy is often used in conjunction with hair, skin, and nail care treatments, massage therapy, acupuncture, reflexology, herbology, chiropractic, hydrotherapy, and other holistic treatments.

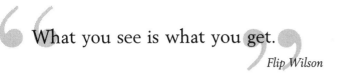

> **What you see is what you get.**
>
> *Flip Wilson*

Ayurvedically Speaking

In Ayurveda, when individuals experience certain imbalances related to their dosha, or mindbody constitution, essential oils can help gently nudge these out-of-balance energies back toward a harmonious state. An unbalanced air principle or energy, with a tendency toward anxiety, irregularity, and restlessness, would do well to select aromatherapies based on floral and fruity scents. These aromas can include, but are not limited to, lavender, bergamot, chamomile, marjoram, and geranium. The unbalanced fire principle or energy may find relief from its inclination toward anger, jealousy, impatience, gastrointestinal problems, and heartburn through cooling and sweet aromas. This could include anything from the mint family, jasmine, cedar, ylang-ylang, rose, and sandalwood. For the earth principle or energy gone awry, there is a predisposition for holding on to things, such as weight or relationships. The best aromas to reverse these effects would be anything stimulating and spicy, like eucalyptus, rosemary, camphor, and sage.

Be the Visionary— Our Sense of Sight

Enlightenment, intuition, meditation, creative visualization, seeing through the mind's eye—these previously covered elements are indeed integral parts of sight. As we continue our journey toward connecting with inner vision and voice, I would like to now take the concept of sight even further. Keep your eyes wide open. You're about to get some captivating insights into creating better balance and healing within the mindbody physiology—for yourself as well as your clients.

See the Beauty in Everyone

As beauty professionals, we are keenly tuned in to how external appearance creates specific impressions or emotional responses. As the old say-

> The Real Voyage of Discovery consists not in
> seeking new landscapes, but in having new eyes.
>
> *Marcel Proust*

ing goes, "What you see is what you get." Even our day-to-day language in the salon or spa mirrors the connection between sight and judgment. For instance, it's not a layered bob, it's a fresh look. Other labels include a modern look, a fashionable look, a sexy look, a traditional look, a care-free look, a sporty look, a rough look, and, yes, even a grunge look. We see how a soccer mom generally has a different look and psyche from the fast-track dot-com diva; the bohemian college student projects a different image from the law firm intern. While these looks refer to one's outward appearance—face, hair, clothing, posture, even mannerisms—they could also mirror a person's spiritual self—life philosophies, values, and expec-tations. We as interpreters, as dream-weavers, play a vital role in help-ing clients present their external countenance in a way that reflects both their physical and emotional selves. You are a creator of visions, repre-senting both inner and outer beauty.

We accomplish this mighty feat in several ways. First and foremost, we share our skill set. When a client brings in a photograph of some celebrity, it is up to us to adapt that look to the individual's hair condi-tion, length, texture, and density, as well as the client's skin, eyes, face shape, and overall body shape. Second, we share our inner sight. As beau-ty professionals, we have the ability to see inherent beauty in each per-son, bringing it gloriously and blissfully outward. Resist the temptation to label or judge others based on outward appearance alone. Be part of, not separate from, a client's desire —be it conscious or subconscious—to holistically unify body, mind, and spirit. You have the power to see a per-son's individual beauty and, indeed, to help the entire world see it.

See the Light

And God said, "Let there be light." With this, we gained the ability to perceive color, shape, and texture. Our eyes work in such a systematic and routine manner, it is easy to forget the miracle of it all.

So how does the miracle of sight occur? How are others literally able to see the visions we create? Our eyes gather light, much like a camera. When we look at something, the retina shoots neurons off to the brain, floating these neurons along an electrochemical stream. The visual cortex

> **"** Our spectrum of consciousness is not separate from the spectrum of light. **"**
>
> *Denise Linn*, Sacred Space

in the brain takes this information and makes sense of it. This allows you to define and label who or what it is that you're seeing. And indeed, some suggest that 70 percent of all sensory information is taken in through the eyes—where a large number of sense receptors are clustered. This may also be one of the reasons that a quarter of our nutritional intake goes toward feeding our visual apparatus.

See the Beauty in Eye Care

Our vision is indeed priceless! Look around you right now. Do a "360." Realize the amazing and wonderful gift that you have in being able to visually take in your world. Do not take your vision for granted. Eyestrain, stress, exposure to environmental toxins, lack of exercise, inadequate or inappropriate nutritional intake, and simply neglect can over time lead to large and small woes—like presbyopia, glaucoma, cataracts, and macular degeneration. Yes, some of these conditions have genetic components, but this only means that you need to be even more diligent in caring for your eyes.

One of your eyes' most common foes is strain. From an Ayurvedic standpoint, the absolutely best remedy for eyestrain would be to reduce stress, meditate, and relax by taking in only the most pleasant of sights. This last one is such a wonderful affirmation—today I will protect my eyes by seeing only pleasant sights. Okay, this may be impossible within the parameters of our daily 24-hour routine, but as you take your after-lunch walk, commute home, or prepare the evening meal, try making it a point to see only beautiful things. Eventually, I promise, you will run out of common, conventionally attractive sights and begin finding beauty in the most unexpected or unusual places! For instance, as I was preparing dinner last night, I found the red pepper on my cutting board particularly appealing and beautiful.

You also want to concentrate on certain daily eye care practices. Take care to rest your eyes, hydrate them with natural tears as needed, use only the most natural products in and around the eyes, and reduce exposure to chemical pollutants. Have your eyes checked at least once a year by a qualified ophthalmologist, or eye doctor. Exercise your eyes by consciously blinking, rotating them, and alternately focusing on close and then distant objects. And do consider programmed vision therapy, or eye calisthenics, to maintain your eyesight or if you find your vision worsening.

When it comes to eye exercise, the muscle that surrounds the eye's lens (the ciliary muscle) as well as the muscles that surround the eyeball (the extraocular muscles) should be routinely moved in different directions.

If you actively care for your eyes through exercise, they'll work more efficiently and exhibit less deterioration with age. So many of us take a passive approach to our eyes, simply relying on corrective lenses to solve vision problems. See the resource section for more details on vision therapy.

> In Chinese medicine, the eyes are said to be nourished by the liver. The liver meridian runs through the tissues surrounding the eyes and brings life force energy to this entire area. Many of the toxins that we take in are filtered through our liver. Therefore, it is essential that you eat as healthily as possible to support the liver's vital function—to process toxins that we are exposed to.
>
> Milk thistle is one of the very best herbs to detoxify the system and support liver function in particular. Also, as a preventative measure against glaucoma and cataracts and to protect your eyes' general health, reduce your intake of saturated fat and cholesterol, which can block the tiny vessels surrounding the eyes, thus creating arteriosclerosis.

Healthy Lighting

We humans need to see the light. Literally. When certain individuals do not get enough light, they can suffer dearly. This is tied to our circadian rhythms, and pertains particularly to individuals who miss out on daylight by working the night shift. Suffering through rainy days and jet lag can also bring on light-deprivation woes. At the most serious level, certain individuals who do not get enough daylight (especially during winter months when daylight hours diminish, or in northern latitudes where darkness prevails for lengthy periods) are afflicted with a condition called S.A.D.—seasonal affective disorder. This can cause excessive fatigue, irritability, and depression. Exposing oneself to very bright light in a light box can treat the condition. These boxes may be purchased in specialty stores or catalogs or through your physician.

So you can see how important it is to get up with the sun, do as much as possible during normal daylight hours, and let your body enjoy plenty of natural light. Natural light helps normalize your adrenal function and more specifically your levels of cortisol (the stress hormone). It also triggers essential physiological processes involving the nervous system and the endocrine system. In addition, it greatly enhances metabolization of vitamin D, the sunshine vitamin, which stimulates the absorption of calcium.

Bringing your life into rhythm with the ebb and flow of natural light is really pretty straightforward. Perform as many of your daily activities as possible in natural or full-spectrum lighting. Try to get at least 10 to 15 minutes of sunlight every day. And here's an F.Y.I.: yogis say that gazing at a full moon strengthens your eyesight as well as your heart. So, go commune with the man in the moon!

Give Yourself the Full Spectrum

Consider installing full-spectrum lighting where you live and work. Full-spectrum lighting, also called natural-spectrum lighting, closely resembles daylight. Studies show that people, pets, and plants all do better under full-spectrum lighting. Its richer, whiter light brings out the truest colors in your surroundings, eases eyestrain, reduces fatigue, and can actually help improve your mood. Personally, I would recommend that every salon and spa have full-spectrum lighting. The resulting benefits are invaluable!

What is Melatonin?

Melatonin is a hormone produced by the pineal gland in the center of the brain. It has been linked to changes in mood, behavior, sleep patterns, fatigue, performance, and our biological rhythms. Light and darkness, temperature, and other factors affect natural levels of melatonin. If you believe your body is running low on melatonin, talk to your doctor about a melatonin supplement.

Visualize Beauty

Just as we humans tend to associate feelings with aromas (think aromatherapy), we also attach feelings to sights. In other words, how you perceive an image can have a dramatic impact on how you react to subsequent views of this image or memories of it.

Having traveled the world, I have some amazing images stored in the software of my mindbody physiology. Recalling these sights brings on a variety of feelings. If a particular image in your mind's eye elicits good feelings, then by all means, go to this place often through creative visualization. A pristine, pastoral image can induce relaxation and serenity. Familiar images can bring on a sense of peace and comfort. Imagining something you've never even seen before can create a sense of expansiveness and exhilaration. And disturbing imagery can make one feel stressed, depressed, or ill at ease.

It should come as no surprise when I tell you that the violence we see through various news media has been linked to negative actions and feelings. Dr. Andrew Weil, a renowned physician at the forefront of integrative medicine, strongly suggests that everyone go on a news fast every so often—separating oneself from the war, famine, and various other atrocities going on internationally. I've done this on numerous occasions, and I find it very therapeutic and gratifying.

Think about the environment that you travel through every day. How does it affect you? Is it cluttered, sloppy, and chaotic, or is it clean, fresh, streamlined, and potent—ripe for your creativity. Remember that your environment is filled with energy. It should be a nourishing environment, vibrating with energy that allows you to transform, enliven, and vitalize every moment of every day. Take pride in creating an environment that surrounds you with this type of transformative energy.

Do an inventory of your workspace. Do you see and thus feel beauty in this space? If not, consider keeping a fresh flower in a simple bud vase. Make certain that your equipment is dazzlingly clean. Don't let anything fall into disrepair. Consider the colors that surround you.

Jot down a few beautiful sights in your work area, sights that please not only you but your clients:

_____

_____

_____

_____

_____

_____

_____

_____

_____

_____

Now write down a few insightful ways to beautify your work area, whether this means making repairs or updates or adding simple joyful touches.

_____

_____

_____

_____

_____

_____

_____

_____

_____

_____

Color Your World

In the spa world, many have integrated the concept of color therapy, also called chromatherapy, into their services. This type of therapy is used to maintain or change bodily vibrations through colored light, color-therapy massage, or hydrotherapy treatments. Of course, there is also the matter of how color in the spa or salon environment influences energy flow and activity throughout this space. We'll talk about this at greater length in a moment, but for now let's just say that color—regardless of intensity—has great power.

Studies prove that color is indeed electromagnetic energy, and it can have a profound effect on our energy fields, creating changes in the mind and body. The colors we see are part of the visible electromagnetic spectrum of light that radiates from the sun. This spectrum ranges from the longest wavelength color, red—vibrating at a low, dense frequency—to the shortest wavelength color, violet, which vibrates at the highest frequency. In between are the colors orange, yellow, green, blue, and indigo. Each of these colors vibrates at its own frequency, and together these colors possess the power to heal and balance us on many levels. This is due to the fact that we sense color vibration not only through our vision but also through all the physical systems and organs in our bodies. Everything responds to these color frequencies. This is why color therapy can have a profound effect on us, creating balance and helping healing take place.

So now let's take a closer look at the power of color. As I define each color's capacity to affect us, notice how I relate it back to the chakra system, which we discussed in Chapter Three, "Beauty in Mind, Body, and Spirit." To refresh your memory, this ancient Hindu concept relates to the seven energy centers found within each individual—the chakras. Each chakra, or center, is a vortex of energy, a spiritual opening in the body where subtle energies may enter and leave. Chakras process subtle energy and convert it into chemical, hormonal, and cellular changes in the body. The chakras act as doorways to our consciousness, allowing ethereal energy to become physical, and physical energy to return to the ethereal realm.

To positively affect the chakras, surround yourself with your appropriate colors—wear these colors, eat these colors, and breathe these colors into your body to affect healing. Before we get down to the nitty-gritty, remember this *synopsis:* reds, oranges, and yellows are stimulating, giving energy and strength. Greens and blues are cooling, cleansing and balancing. Purple induces lightness of being and enhances intuition.

As you read on and become more familiar with each color, think of ways to integrate more or less of a particular color into your world. For instance, if you feel you need more blue, eat blueberries, wear blue jeans, look at the blue sky, gaze at the indigo night sky, paint your walls blue, and at the very least accessorize your surroundings with blue. Finally, when you creatively visualize, color the imagery you see with lots of healing blue!

Red is traditionally the color of the Root Chakra, located at the base of the spine. In its highest manifestation, the color red expresses divine will because this chakra is at the center of our survival. Red vitalizes and stimulates all bodies. It is responsible for a sound physical body, since it affects our circulatory system, digestion, and elimination. When these systems are not working in harmony, you can feel fatigued. Red helps maintain color in the skin and gives energy to nerve tissue and bone marrow. A lack of red can manifest as abscesses, anemia, blood disorders, cancer, insomnia, as well as circulatory, digestive, and heart problems.

Orange is traditionally the color of the Navel/Hara Chakra, or the center of fertility—both creative and sexual. Orange expresses wisdom in its greatest form and gives energy and strength to the sex organs. Orange can also relieve depression brought on by insecurity and fear, and it can build self-esteem through creative and intellectual stimulation. Some illnesses associated with a lack of orange's vibratory energy are asthma, epilepsy, female reproductive problems, kidney ailments, and mental instability.

Yellow is traditionally the color of the Solar Plexus Chakra, and it expresses divine intellect, as it is in this chakra that you form opinions based on all subtle energetic levels of sensation. These sensations and your reactions to them allow you to develop a strong sense of self. Yellow promotes understanding and intelligence and helps energy rise to the crown chakra for spiritual realization. Yellow works with the body as a purifier and cleanser. It illuminates and inspires, allowing your higher consciousness to develop. It promotes all forms of mental activity. It also stimulates optimism. Some illnesses associated with a lack of yellow energy include skin diseases, heartburn, hemorrhoids, diabetes, and impotence.

Green is traditionally the color of the Heart Chakra, and is the universal color for healing. It is quite balancing and cleansing and brings energy and feelings of happiness to our center of unconditional love—the heart. Green creates a condition of well-being and stability on all levels, helping to overcome anxiety, intolerance, and irritability. Work with the color green if you are challenged with any of the following: cancer, miscarriage, nervous disorders, blood pressure and circulatory problems, or heart disease, as well as gall bladder and kidney stones.

Blue is traditionally the color of the Throat Chakra, and it expresses truth, since the fifth chakra deals with outward expression of self—the way in which we tactfully and elegantly communicate with others. Blue works primarily with the energies of the throat in that it gives expression to creativity in a way that reflects the inner self. Bring more blue into your mindbody physiology if you find yourself challenged by problems related to the eyes, ears, nose, and throat, as well as irritability, laryngitis, tonsillitis, and sexual dysfunction.

Indigo is traditionally the color of the Third Eye Chakra, and it expresses enlightenment. This is the ability to see things as they really are, thus promoting clarity in thought as well as tolerance. Indigo purifies the bloodstream and mental processes. It also promotes unity and stability of your higher subtle bodies. It has even been used to induce local, and in certain cases total, anesthesia. Lack of indigo can be related to mental stability, lung ailments, menopausal problems, sterility, delirium, and eye, ear, and nose problems.

Violet is traditionally the color of the Crown Chakra, and it can create incredible lightness of being in the body while also helping to open the doors of perception. It expresses metamorphosis as well as devotion, while also enhancing inspirational energies and intuition. Violet encourages a dedication to higher truths and ideals by blending the love in the color red with the truth and devotion in the color blue. Bring more violet into your life if you find yourself challenged by scalp problems, blood ailments, tumors, vertigo, concussion, delusional disorders, and convulsions.

I have given you only the briefest of overviews here relating to color therapy and its proven beneficial effects on our mindbody physiology. Please take it upon yourself to study further this intriguing and provocative subject.

In Ayurveda, the use of color therapy is seen as an important sensory modulation technique to bring about nurturing balance. Warm and/or muted colors can calm an anxious air constitution (gold, muted orange or yellow, deep purple, indigo). Cool, soothing colors can pacify a fire constitution (light blues or greens), and warm, stimulating bright colors can invigorate an earth constitution (bright reds, yellow, orange).

> **" Let us be silent that we may hear
> the whispers of God. "**
>
> *Ralph Waldo Emerson*

The Sense of Sound—
All Is Rhythm

Primal sound is everywhere as a divine vibration. The ancient Egyptians called the universal vibratory energies the words of their gods; the Pythagoreans of Greece called these energies the music of the spheres; and the ancient Chinese knew them as the celestial energies of perfect harmony. Around us and within us, every atom in the universe is indeed vibrating. The cosmic symphony is everywhere, but we do need to tune in. Mystics, shamans, priests, and healers have heard and helped others to hear this symphony for millennia. Hence the long and powerful history of mantras, chanting, toning, drumming, and music, all used to access the balancing and healing nature of sound.

When you meditate with a mantra or to the rhythm of your breath, you seek communion with the divine. When you tone or chant your body into attunement, you find peace. And when you drum you seek to restore harmonic patterns of vibration that are in tune with universal vibration— the cosmic symphony.

We've explored how matter is vibrating energy or energy in motion. That is, energy on the verge of becoming matter, and matter on the verge of becoming energy. How we experience sound or vibration, whether in silence or of the audible variety, can have a tremendous impact on our thoughts—since thoughts are vibrating energy—as well as on our ability to communicate with others. To truly hear another, we must first develop an inner silence. This connects us to our truest nature. When you come from this place, you are more able to participate in meaningful communication.

I understand that this may seem somewhat far out for some of you, however it is very real. It is what the ancient Rishis tell us in their Vedic texts from over 5,000 years ago. And it is also what modern quantum physics and modern science tell us. Many music and sound therapies exist today, using music and/or sound to help clients attain therapeutic goals—objectives that can be mental, physical, emotional, social, or spiritual in nature.

> *God gave man two ears, but only one mouth, that he might hear twice as much as he speaks.*
>
> *Epictetus the Stoic*

Meaningful Communication

To listen actively and really hear what another person says is not only good for your personal well-being but it is also a highly regarded skill in our particular profession. A good listener is able to repeat back everything the other person says—not parrotlike but rather with an understanding for the feelings behind the words. This does not mean that you need to immediately get every person's deepest meaning. No, it means that a good listener hears when it's time to ask questions— interesting ones. A good listener *hears* the missing information, or senses a need for more information in order to successfully complete the communication. When you ask questions, however, make certain you phrase your query so that you can truly receive information. Ask "How did your haircut work for you since I saw you last time?" instead of "Do you want your hair cut the same way as last time?" And then really listen to the response. Remember, communication is an art form that can be perfected.

Vibrational Nutrition

We take in sound vibrations from our surroundings. This energy passes through the middle ear, creating waves in the fluid-filled inner ear, the cochlea. These sound waves move tiny hairs in the cochlea, triggering nerve cells to send electrical energy onward to the brain. Our nervous system then translates these sound impulses as pleasant (serving to relax the body) or unpleasant (causing the body to feel stress). Pleasant sounds, particularly pleasurable music, can enhance our immune system activity, with white blood cells picking up this agreeable beat as they flow through the body via the lymphatic system. You produce endorphins and bathe yourself with joy-inducing neurotransmitters as you listen to enjoyable sounds.

It is now proven beyond a shadow of a doubt that sound can have amazing effects on delicate cells, tissues, and organs. Vibrating sounds form patterns and create resonating energy fields around us. We absorb these energies, and they in turn can alter our breath, pulse, blood pressure, muscle tension, skin temperature, and produce other physical changes. Also consider this—we absorb good vibrations through our skin and bones as well as our eardrums. Is this what they mean by Surround Sound?

Naturally, everyone has a different perception of pleasant versus disturbing sounds. What one person sees as symphonic genius, another sees as discordant junk. Pulsing hip-hop may help one person move to the groove and get work done with efficiency and style, while for someone else this type of music can sound like fingernails scratching across a chalkboard, setting them on edge and making them irritable. Honor your preferences as well as those of others. In the salon or spa where you work, modulate the musical vibe, selections, and decibel levels to please as many clients as possible. (Yes, it is true, you cannot please all the people all the time, but you can achieve some general agreement!) If associates and clients have widely different preferences, perhaps you can designate one day and/or night a week for "techno-ambient grooves," another time period for "operetta delights," and yet another for jazz greats. Maybe dedicate a night to the "King"—Elvis, that is. Post your musical menu at the front desk, on your website, or in your newsletter, and encourage clients to book appointments according to their favorite beat. Make every beauty service a true experience. In a culture where we look for new and different experiences, this could set your business apart from and above the rest.

The Research Is In

- In one study, conducted at Baltimore's St. Agnes Hospital, patients in critical care units listened to classical music. Half an hour of music produced the same effect as ten milligrams of Valium.
- A study at Michigan State University found that listening to music for fifteen minutes increased people's interleukin-1 levels more than 10 percent. Interleukins are proteins that provide cellular protection against AIDS and cancer.
- In one remarkable study, conducted at Bulgaria's Academy of Sciences and Sofia Medical Institute, students who listened to string instruments improved their learning abilities. The subjects learned complex tasks in a fraction of the time that it would have normally taken; a semester's training was reduced to a few hours.

> I want to sing like birds sing, not worrying
> who hears or what they think.
>
> *Rumi*

- In Norway, music therapy was used for children with severe physical and mental disabilities. They were immersed in a "musical bath" that reduced muscle tension and, in patients suffering from spastic conditions, increased their range of movement in the spine, hips, legs, and arms.
- Studies out of the University of Washington found that the accuracy of copy editors increased 21.3 percent when they listened to light classical music.

Sound Advice

Breathing, mantras, chanting, drumming, the sounds of nature, and music are all ways in which we can bring ourselves to a place of wholeness. Healing sounds create a resonance within your nervous system that balances your mindbody physiology. Brain-wave coherence is optimized, and healing chemicals as well as hormones are released within your body when you are exposed to healing sound.

Definitely worth noting are the sounds of nature, which tend to have a very pacifying effect on us. Think about how you feel when listening to early-morning bird melodies, evening cricket chirps, the lonely call of the loon, a haunting wolf's cry, wind rustling through the trees, a thunderstorm, or a gentle rain . . . these are all sounds that enliven and rejuvenate us. (By the way, many of nature's most wonderful sounds are available on CD, if you don't think a loon or wolf will be visiting your neighborhood anytime soon.) This earth is vibrating with life-force energy, and this energy is transmitted to us through the music of nature. Nature conducts one of the most magnificent symphonies that one could ever hear, and as I've said before, we're an expression of this symphony.

Musical Notes

Music has been shown to have biochemical effects on the body, which only makes sense since rhythm is integral to music as well as to our bodies. Think biorhythm—the innate, cyclical clock by which all biological systems function. The body's biorhythm conducts all bodily functions, including respiration, circulation, regulation of fluid levels, digestion, and elimination of toxins. Music can calm, soothe, or energize these functions and processes. Music can also reduce pain, tension, and the need for medication. Consider these facts—proven as much through practical life as scientific research:

- Sedative music lowers heart and respiration rates along with blood pressure. Sedative music, slow in tempo and with a quality close to the human voice, tends to feature violins and flutes, as opposed to horns and percussion. Or, think folk music! Digital and/or certain ethereal, otherworldly styles of music can also be quite sedating.
- Repetition can be very soothing. Look for CDs with chanting or drumming set to music.
- Stimulating music—Mozart (especially touted for the energy-balancing qualities of his compositions) and Vivaldi are excellent examples—can be quite liberating or exhilarating.

Easy listening, opera, country/western, acid jazz, blues, rock and roll, flamenco, alternative house—all these different music styles can guide your mood and your emotional state. Listen to and use them all, using a selection at a given moment to either reflect your present mood or lead your mood to where you wish it to be. For instance, you may prefer a dynamic beat with higher volume levels as you get dressed for the day, perhaps soothing and fluid sounds with a moderate tempo during afternoon breaks, and easy, ambient rhythms in the evening.

The right music can also help ease you into a form of meditation. Sit comfortably, eyes closed, and breathe in smoothly and deeply while taking in your musical choice. Get into the music with your entire mind, body, and soul. Whether it is sedating or stimulating in nature, follow your instincts when it comes to the music and let the rhythm move you—whether emotionally or physically. I enjoy playing music that relaxes me, and I also enjoy, when the time is right, music that gets my body going, as I perform what can only be called free-form dance. Do whatever feels right and become one with the music. This is all a form of self-healing—physical activity coming together with music to energize or soothe the body, mind, and soul.

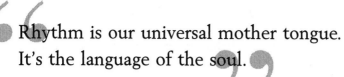

Rhythm is our universal mother tongue.
It's the language of the soul.

Gabrielle Roth

Here are only a few of the impressions we receive from different musical styles. Much depends on our environment and our own unique mindbody physiology. I've offered a few specific composers or titles that create certain impressions, but your favorite music shop will be able to supply many more.

- **Gregorian Chant**—Reduces stress and creates a sense of relaxed spaciousness. Excellent for quiet study and meditation.
- **Sacred Music**—Brings you into present-moment awareness. Creates feelings of deep peace and spiritual awareness. Can also help us in rising above and releasing pain.
- **Romantic Music**—Emphasizes feelings of love and compassion. The Romantic composers include Chopin, Liszt, Schubert, Schumann, and Tchaikovsky.
- **Rock and Roll**—Music by the Beatles, the Rolling Stones, R.E.M., Limp Bizkit, Blink 182, Elvis Presley, the Grateful Dead: it can all stir the passions, stimulate us to move, release tension, relieve pain, and reduce the effects of other loud or disturbing sounds in our environment. Do note, however, that if we are not in the mood to be energetically entertained, this music can create tension, stress, and pain in our bodies.
- **Jazz, Blues, Dixieland, Soul, Calypso, and Reggae**—Any one of these musical styles can uplift and inspire, release deep joy as well as sadness, and affirm our oneness with humanity.

Drumming Circle

Once confined to aboriginal tribes, Native American rituals, or loin-clothed men's circles, drumming has entered the mainstream as a sound therapy. It is used by indigenous tribes around the world to effect profound transformation and healing. Drumming at a certain frequency brings one to what in shamanism is referred to as "non-ordinary" reality. This is where we find our power, and where soul retrieval takes place. It is where we tap deeply into the core of universal energy. It is where we shapeshift mentally, physically, emotionally, and spiritually.

I belong to a drumming circle, and together, for several hours once a month, we create the most amazing and vital energy. In this process, the sound of our drums catches us in its spiral and catapults us into a most transformative and breathtaking experience. It just plain brings everyone together into one big, smiley, interactive experience.

There are many exceptional tapes and CDs to help you enjoy and partake of this healing and transformative therapy. Or you may want to invest in your own drum! Do also consider other forms of instrumental sound to bring harmony into your world, such as a Tibetan "singing" bowl, bells, gongs, rattles, and wind chimes. All of these healing sounds may be used in your personal as well as professional environment to anoint, clear, and energize your space.

Drum Up Your Immunity

It may not sound like medicine, but rhythmic drumming may do wonders for your health. Researchers from the Mind-Body Wellness Center in Meadville, Pennsylvania, and the Center for Neuroimmunology at the Loma Linda University School of Medicine conducted studies where levels of immune system markers in the blood were measured before and after drumming. Those who performed group drumming, an activity that combines guided imagery with several drumming styles, showed increased immune activity. Drumming therapy is already practiced in the U.S. as a supportive treatment for a variety of diseases, including cancer, cardiovascular disease, chronic lung diseases, diabetes, and asthma. If you are unable to find a group drumming program in your area, the people at a local music store may know about such programs or may be able to help you get your own started.

As a matter of fact, how about forming a drumming circle at the salon or spa where you work? Start with one evening and extend an open invitation to clients as well as associates. Who knows, it could become a regular affair! Doesn't that sound great?

You Don't Say

Our voices deliver their own mellifluous melodies outward into the world. I fondly remember my mother singing around the house when I was growing up. Go ahead and hum, sing, shout from the mountaintop—all effective ways to make memories as well as cleanse and strengthen the voice. As we age, the vocal cords and larynx can begin to lose resiliency and tone. This doesn't have to be the case. Whether speaking, singing, toning, or chanting, let yourself be heard and accentuate your vocal resonance.

Voice Training

People really do remember your voice and can be attracted or repulsed by it. It puts out a certain vibe. Tone, pitch, cadence, and accent, combined with body language, appearance, vocabulary, and content, all combine to make for speech. What an education it was when I listened to my voice in a recording. Consider your own voice. If it is not what you wish to hear, consider the following:

- Speak slowly. This causes people to listen more closely.
- Breathe diaphragmatically. It helps produce a clear, rhythmic sound.
- Stand up straight. This puts less strain on your vocal cords, opens air passages, and allows you to feel more natural when speaking. An added benefit is the confident body language you communicate.
- Practice singing scales, from low to high and back again. This gives you a wider and more flexible vocal range. Your voice will sound more harmonious and smooth.
- Recite all the consonants, out loud, every day. This creates better resonance and builds strong throat muscles.
- Project your voice. Visualize your voice hitting a point on the wall. Move farther away and closer, adjusting your voice as you move. Remember, projection is not shouting.
- Use pauses. This can make a huge difference in the cadence of your speech.
- Inject passion into your voice. Be enthusiastic, but you must really know as well as believe what you're saying, of course.

Toning

Toning, an ancient practice gaining newfound popularity, allows the body to find its own balance, and thus release stress, balance brain waves, slow down respiration, and actually give the body a massage from the inside out. It works through sustained vibration (like that of a tuning fork) that resonates through the entire body for a dramatic impact on our energies.

In toning, you sing a vowel sound at a certain comfortable pitch for a prolonged period of time. Vibrations reverberate through the body, affecting it in profound ways, with different sounds working different ways. Lower "aah" sounds allow the body to relax. Higher "eee" sounds stimulate the brain and wake you up. The rest of the story is very simple; take in a deep diaphragmatic breath, and let loose with your tone. Try varying the intensities of tone, sound, and pitch. For best results, try toning every day for at least 5 minutes per session.

Chanting

Chanting is similar to toning, but instead you chant a mantra or primordial sound. Try the Sanskrit word "Om" (also spelled "Aum"). Hindus and Buddhists believe this sound to be the manifestation of a person's spiritual self. It is the hymn of the universe, evoking the beginning of time, the cosmic truth, the infinity of being. I find this to be one of my most resonant sounds for chanting, and I end my meditations with it.

Toxic Sound

Sound levels can be hazardous to our hearing, and in this instance *sound* refers to noise, and *hazard* applies to physical as well as psychological harm. It is important to take precautions against excessive noise. You can save yourself untold millions of inner ear cells plus a lot of aggravation and tension.

If you are around loud noises for extended periods, wear earplugs. They are comfortable to wear, made of form-fitting foam, and come in funky as well as conventional colors. Don't worry, you can hear just fine while wearing ear plugs. They only mute high decibels or aggressive noises that can inflict hearing damage.

When I speak of physical as well as psychological harm, one of the biggest concerns is that overexposure to loud noise can destroy your ability to hear frequencies above 3,000 cycles per second. This, in turn, robs you of your capacity to enjoy healing music. Optimally, we hear frequencies ranging from 20 to 20,000 cycles per second, almost ten octaves; without this capability, music sounds like mush. You will miss out on much of the healing energy transmitted by the higher harmonics.

On a purely psychological level, noise undermines our mental and creative energy. It's distracting, since clamor demands a series of cognitive decisions, taking us away from our work or focus. Perhaps you're trying to consult with your client, but blaring music makes communication difficult. Or maybe you're trying to enjoy a meal, but a blabbering tableside television is directing your attention away from the peas and carrots. Even a churning air conditioner can prevent you from getting a good night's sleep. All these little things can cumulatively cause problems. The solution may be to neutralize the noise. Many options exist.

How Loud Is Loud?

The Occupational Safety and Health Administration has set noise limits of 90 decibels for eight hours of work and 95 decibels for four hours, but some experts feel that these levels are unacceptable. They contend that if you need to raise your voice to be heard by someone three feet away (background noise at 45 to 50 decibels), this environment is hazardous to your hearing. A few sounds with their decibel levels are listed below as a reference. Keep in mind that if you go up 10 decibels, you double the loudness of a sound!

- Wind rustling through the leaves—20 decibels
- Normal conversation—50–60 decibels
- Hair dryer—60–80 decibels
- Crowded city street—90 decibels
- Stereo at full volume—120 decibels
- Jet takeoff—130–140 decibels

Anti-Noise Technology

The salon can be a noisy environment . . . doors opening and closing, phones ringing, music or talk radio going, many voices mixing it up, blow dryers whooshing, water running—the sounds of life! Depending on the materials used to construct and decorate your work environment, these sounds can be quite intense.

Many companies now manufacture and/or sell products to quiet noise levels and improve acoustics in a building. These products blend into the environment and go a long way toward moderating "noisy" atmospheres. One of the best resources for noise-reduction products is www.noisesuppression.com.

Here are a few more suggestions:

- Wear foam earplugs. They suppress noise that can distract and irritate you.
- Look for electronic and home appliances that have the lowest possible decibel rating.
- Decorate your environment with soft surfaces like drapery, upholstery, and carpeting, which all absorb noise instead of allowing it to bounce around.
- Install baffles or panels that may be inconspicuously placed along walls, hanging from the ceiling, or under chairs to absorb reverberating sounds.
- Install double-glazed windows.
- If possible, avoid working or living in the midst of a major noise source, such as an airport, truck route, freeway, or busy intersection. Of course, this takes forethought before renting or buying, but it's an important point to put on your list of considerations.

Sound Health

In addition to reducing damage-inducing noise levels and increasing our exposure to soothing sounds, here are a few more common-sense but often overlooked ways to protect your ears:

- Eat a low-fat, low-cholesterol diet. A high-fat diet clogs and hardens the arteries, impairing the flow of nutrient-rich blood throughout the body—including to the inner ear.
- Get regular exercise to improve blood circulation.
- If experiencing any degree of hearing loss, have your hearing checked by a medical professional. Your problem may be something as simple as a build-up of wax, or it could be something more serious. Other hearing problems to immediately look into include a ringing in the ears, vertigo, and TMJ—temporomandibular joint problems.
- Consider using your cell phone less or consider putting an electromagnetic phone shield on it. A cell phone sends out electromagnetic frequencies that travel into the brain through the ear canal, and there is some concern that these frequencies have potential cancer-causing effects.

- Be extremely gentle when cleansing the ear and ear canal area. Also, make sure to include the ears as part of your delicious self-massage, massaging gently with a small amount of oil. Pull on the earlobe, then delicately massage with the thumb and index finger around the entire ear lobe. Use the index finger tip to massage behind the ear as well as the inner ear. This simple process relaxes the muscles and joints through the jaw and neck. It stimulates many organs and glands, especially those that affect the skin.

A Final Harmonious Note

While our ears are the sense organs for *hearing* sound, our mouths are the sense organs for *delivering* sound. The mouth, lips, teeth, gums, and tongue are quite sensual parts of the body. The tongue allows us to communicate with the world. Our lips are a provocative extension of the mucous membranes found inside the mouth. Our teeth express our happiness and pleasure when we flash those pearly whites. Lavish loving attention on your mouth. Slather organic balms on your lips, eat nourishing foods, meticulously cleanse your mouth, massage your gums every day with sesame oil, and sing a happy tune!

Naturally, as beauty and wellness professionals, we also want to pay special attention to oral hygiene. I'm all for thoroughly enjoying a meal, but it is not fair to ask our clients to share the experience as well . . . an hour later in the form of garlic or stale breath.

I've heard it said that the longer we keep our natural teeth, the longer our life span. Holding on to your original teeth is intricately involved with gum health. Genetics aside, problems with teeth and gums are generally rooted in a lack of good care. Poor oral hygiene can cause some fairly major problems. And now there is even more incentive to brush and floss. Regular flossing for at least one to two minutes a day is one of the best preventatives for gum disease, which can cause oral bacteria to enter your bloodstream and potentially narrow blood vessels, increase blood clots, and put you at greater risk for a heart attack. Love your heart. Brush and floss at least twice a day. Also, do visit your dentist at least once a year (twice is even better!) for regular check-ups and cleanings. Couple this with maintaining your optimal water intake. And keep natural breath mints or drops on hand at your work station (very important!).

Fresh, vital, and beautiful, the language of our senses is universal, and it is revealed to us in precious details. May your senses gather you and bring you home—where you may experience your truest self.

Notes:

Chapter Eight

A Conclusion That Marks the Beginning

Holistic beauty care takes flight in an environment where a full menu of beauty and wellness services is offered, services that provide for a nurturing balance between mind, body, and spirit. It is an environment where your own beauty and wellness knowledge comes forth and flows outward to create an experience of wholeness for yourself, your clients, and your fellow beauty professionals. You understand from a higher, expanded level of consciousness what your incredible healing abilities are and how they can make people feel good. And you feel your own power, your own beauty, your own wholeness. Every thought you have, every action you take, serves to maintain the exquisite flow of life-force energy through and around you.

Holistic beauty is also about opening your mind to infinite possibilities, thinking far beyond job definitions learned in school and reaching upward toward professional potential—total career consciousness. Today, holistic beauty includes manicures, massages, and mammograms. Yes, mammograms—and osteoporosis screenings, too. Today it is possible to enter a single building and get your hair done, move on to dream analysis with a psychotherapist, then finish your visit with a yoga class or a seminar on raw foods, Ayurveda, or perhaps low-fat cooking. At one salon, clients can book back-to-back appointments with a colorist and a chiropractor. At another, a plastic surgeon gives collagen injections while a podiatrist waits to treat a variety of foot ailments. At a spa I know of, they're integrating health, beauty, and fitness by offering breathing techniques as part of many treatments. Yet another establishment provides haircuts as well as nutritional counseling and regular Friday-night Satsangs. The Sanskrit word for a gathering of people to share the truth, a Satsang is a sacred assembly that can include spiritual discussion, music, chanting, meditation, and refreshments. It may be a new word to you now, but it's becoming quite popular.

And there are more educational meetings going on, for the beauty professional and beauty guest alike. One spa holds weekly laughing club gatherings. Many spas now offer meals served by an on-site chef. There are stress and weight management offerings, as well as therapeutic touch, Thai massage, Reiki, acupuncture, Pilates and yoga, meditation rooms—they are all part of total beauty and wellness, and they are all being offered at salons and spas. The haircut is quickly becoming part of an enlightenment process rather than a monthly item on the to-do list.

If you are not presently part of all this enlightenment but wish you were, seek out establishments that foster such environments. Or you could help create this attitude toward integrated services in your own spa or salon. You could become the community's premier holistic spa, salon, or energy center—if you dream it, visualize it. Then go manifest it.

Just as health, beauty, and fitness professionals work side by side these days, many beauty professionals are individually offering expanded services. For instance, if you are a hairdesigner, you might make it a point to delve into and study skin care. Aside from expanding your services, you may find yourself providing clients with vital insights into critical health issues. Perhaps you spot a mole on a client's neck. You can share your knowledge of moles and recommend that your client see a dermatologist—either one on the premises or a physician you feel comfortable recommending. Other areas where you as a beauty professional or your salon or spa can choose to expand and better serve clients' needs might be liposuction, laser surgery, bikini waxing, and makeup lessons. At the very least, when medically oriented treatments are not offered on the premises, have a rock-solid referral network in place.

Salon and spa websites and newsletters offer a veritable wealth of information about what's happening inside these forward-thinking environments. Constantly updated reports include Q&A's with beauty and wellness professionals, nutritional information and updates, the newest hair silhouettes—you name it, it's being covered. This is true beauty and wellness integration. And this paradigm shift is no fad. Look for more shifting and blending of career definitions and options. Become a visionary. Learn as much as you possibly can to always be flowing along this river of never-ending knowledge. No doubt about it—we are quickly becoming pivotal elements in the healthcare system. The lines between health, fitness, and beauty are blurring as you read. This is the macrocosm—the big picture—of our beauty and wellness universe.

Now for the Microcosm

A galaxy filled with infinite possibilities builds from a million tiny stars. Any one of the blessings I am about to list will bring a nanosecond of peace to yourself, your loved ones, your clients, and your fellow beauty pros. All together or in combination, these singular expressions have the potential to change a life.

Microcosmically speaking, let's look at some of these expressions of holistic beauty. Truly, it comes down to what you give of yourself to each person.

- It could be a smile, a hug, your lightheartedness, or a gentle touch.
- It's the warmth of your hellos and goodbyes to each client.
- It's the serene vibration that emanates from you.
- It's the physical and emotional safety that you extend to a client.
- It's your ability to listen with grace and sensitivity, keenly tuning in to others and finding solutions to their problems.
- It's your ability to speak with honesty, kindness, and genuine concern.
- It's your present-moment awareness, of yourself and the beautiful, sensitive soul sitting in your chair.
- It's your patience.
- It's your non-judgment and understanding.
- It's your unbridled creativity and intuition.
- It's your dedication to the quality of your craft, your attention to every facet, every nuance of your beauty and wellness service.
- It's educating your client about every beautifying step you take throughout a service, and explaining the benefit in each particular step.

- It's the thoroughness you give to educating clients about home maintenance, so they may continue to enjoy the positive energy experienced during a visit with you.
- It's conversation centered on beauty and well-being.
- It's a cut that has been texturized to perfection, allowing hair to fall beautifully and with natural movement.
- It's color that is as natural as possible with minimal upkeep.
  - It's a massage that addresses specific needs, such as muscle relaxation or body alignment, stress reduction, or individual privacy needs.
  - It's how you educate a client about the benefits of massage, explaining what takes place within the mindbody physiology as they receive a nurturing treatment.
    - It's the skin care treatment that is explained simply, yet in depth, so a client can emulate this holistic process at home.
- It's the organic plant oil that you massage into your client's scalp to serve as protection before a chemical service.
- It's the purified water, as well as the organic teas, coffees, juices, and fresh fruit and vegetables you serve clients.
  - It's the floral arrangements throughout your workspace.
    - It's the meditation space and cafe area where you can go to give yourself emotional as well as nutritional respites.
    - It's the natural materials that compose your environment, from the flooring to a trickling waterfall, from the current beauty and wellness publications available for all to the organic art lining the walls.
- It's the reclining shampoo chair that makes a client feel oh so comfortable.
- It's the care given to your work area.
- It's the soothing sights, sounds, and aromas within your environment, void of toxic noise and smells that might offend those who are sensitive or allergic.
- It's the boar-bristle brush you use.
- It's recycling.

- It's your dedication to products that have not been tested on animals and are minimally packaged in order to reduce waste.
- It's the natural fibers that you wear, the certified organic linens that you use, and the certified organic personal care and sanitary products you provide in the ladies' room.

It's Spirit . . . it's your guardian angel . . . it's your mentor watching over you. It's all of this and so much more. Spend a few moments now and reflect on the environment that you work in every day. Reflect on your attitude and approach. Reflect on your fellow beauty pros and your beauty guests. Write down what holistic beauty care means to you. Nontoxic, holistic environments and holistic beauty professionals are going 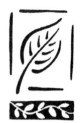 to become the norm, not the exception. Position yourself, your environment, and your services as holistic and nontoxic, aligned with the rhythms of the universe and nurturing of that beautiful flow of life-force energy. Do this and you will have tremendous success, from a spiritual, creative, and financial perspective. You can indeed align yourself with these energies. You simply need to bring this wholly into your consciousness—affirm, visualize, and create this as your reality. The potential is within you. Oliver Wendell Holmes said, "What lies behind us and what lies ahead of us are tiny matters compared to what lies within us."

What holistic beauty care means to me:

_____

_____

_____

_____

_____

_____

_____

_____

Ways I can expand my horizons and raise my consciousness so I can fully participate in the paradigm shift taking place within the beauty profession. These are ways I can align myself with the energies flowing in, through, and around my career—my calling.

_____

_____

_____

_____

_____

_____

_____

_____

_____

_____

Notes:

In Continuation—
The World of Holistic
Beauty Care

> " I am from everlasting the seed of
> eternal life. I am the intelligence
> of the intelligent. I am the beauty
> of the beautiful . . . "
>
> *The Bhagavad Gita*

We've been hanging out together for hundreds of pages—me sharing a portion of my soul, and you, hopefully, getting fully involved. If you take anything away once the last page is read and you close the book, I hope you understand that it all comes down to our being able to experience holistic beauty and bring it into every facet of our work—beginning with ourselves and then flowing outward to all we meet. To accomplish this, we need to come from an exquisite place of whole-ness—a place where body, mind, soul, actions, services, products, and environment all come together in divine synergy.

You hold the magic—the transformative powers—to achieve such synergy. And when you do, you will have successfully ignited that spark we discussed back in Chapter One,

> "I challenge you to a deeper life, and for the sake of those you serve, to seek a stronger bond with your own soul so that you will continually bring new truths to light and help fit others for the living and understanding of these truths."
>
> *A Tibetan master*

"Behold the Beauty Within." Also back at the beginning, I asked you to imagine this tiny spark spiraling outward, casting a beautiful glow upon every thing and every person you see. After all we've been through together, can you now see this image in your mind's eye? Do you see how your own synergy becomes the world's synergy? As healers, shamans, caregivers, *beauty and wellness professionals*, we touch others on so many levels, guiding, teaching, and challenging others to feel as beautiful and whole as possible—to be the very best they can be. As this mighty power begins to radiate outward, let it flow freely toward those you are in communion with and through the environment in which you travel. And remember, this environment is simply an extension of our bodies. See your environment and all living creatures in these terms, and your interactions will constantly serve to strengthen this interconnectedness.

Continuing on the Path

Holistic thought and action comes from a place where you know that interconnectedness—wholeness—is more beautiful, more transformative, more awesome, more powerful, more synergistic than any single part of the whole. We are the ones who create fragmentation and divisiveness, through perceptions, thoughts, and beliefs. These thoughts and beliefs are ours to change. As Buddha said, "We are what we think. All that we are arises with our thoughts. With our thoughts, we make the world."

With that thought, I began the epilogue to this book. Now, however, I see it more as a continuation, or a continuum, if you will. Truly, as stated above, we will all continue on our path from here. There is always something new to learn, some old piece of knowledge to update or some previously asked question to rethink. Synergy is not stagnant. It means union, fellowship, togetherness, communion. Because we live in an ever-changing world, achieving synergy takes daily effort, not only communing with what you already know and believe, but also integrating into your body of knowledge all that is just now rising to the surface in life's river of energy and information, a river that is forever changing, growing, and expanding.

What We've Shared

We've explored much together:

Spiritual communion—where reflection, introspection, meditation, and prayer bring us to a place where beauty, harmony, inspiration, order, and peace deliver us to our higher selves.

Celebration—where we honor the creation of our lives and the fulfillment of our dreams, and where we recognize our losses—whether mourning loved ones or dashed hopes—knowing that there are lessons to be learned here as well.

Integrity and authenticity—where we become our most authentic selves, able to create, realize self-worth, and give meaning to all we do. It is at this point that we begin to share our truest nature with those we are in communion with.

Discernment—where we learn to hear our spirit within, listening to our intuitive wisdom and knowing instinctively how much to take on, take in, or let out. When we acknowledge our own wise judgment, we can enter into relationships and become an effective caregiver, always doing what we can and never making promises to do what we can't.

Interdependence—where we experience community, acceptance, respect, appreciation, support, closeness, trust, understanding, empathy, playfulness, emotional safety, and, yes, love. For those creating their best possible selves, remember that you are never alone. We are all here to help each other in this incredible work. We come and go in each other's lives for a purpose. We are here as guides, students, teachers, and companions.

Your spirituality, your joy in celebration, your integrity and authenticity, your discernment, your interconnectedness—these are all gifts that should be shared. Do it passionately. Put your uniqueness, your spontaneity, your love of life out there. You can do it! It's a matter of deciding that you want to!

> Weapons cannot hurt the Self and fire can never burn him. Untouched is he by drenching waters, untouched is he by parching winds. Beyond the power of sword and fire, beyond the power of waters and winds, the Self is everlasting . . . never changing . . . ever One. Know that he is, and cease from sorrow.
>
> *The Bhagavad Gita*

Tall order, you say? Not when spirit is leading the charge. With spirit at the helm, giving as well as accepting become joyous events. If, however, you reach a point where you have no more to give or you have no need to accept—then perhaps the river has temporarily gone dry. This is not a permanent condition. To know it all is impossible. To have nothing left to share means you've stopped growing. You can tap into the wellspring inside you! Between the riverhead—the source—within and the information flowing freely around us, we could literally go a lifetime and never know it all. You are a channel through which spirit flows. This is continuous and everlasting. You control the flow through your mindfulness and consciousness. The only thing that will never become obsolete is our ability to learn. Now more than ever, we have so many reasons— some might say an obligation—to share what we learn. As beauty and wellness professionals, this directly relates to us.

We have shifted from the materially oriented industrial society of the past to a service-oriented information society; now we are in the process of becoming an experience- and transformation-oriented society and economy. This new orientation means that we can potentially transform our beauty guests' worlds through the experiences we offer them. What's more, our society is slowly becoming more accepting and even expectant of this sharing of experiences between service professionals and their clients.

How do we garner the knowledge that our beauty guests expect us to share with them? We can grow and learn through a variety of channels. One particular channel I want to stress is the World Wide Web. Beauty and wellness information resources abound on the Web, and here we can find endless links to enlightenment. It is one of the most fertile resources for continuing education, as well as providing ties to fellow beauty pros;

information on upcoming seminars; book, video, and magazine reviews; plus a great deal more—all viable channels for yet more information and experiences.

So go out there and choose your dreams, goals, and values; then go forward to plan and enact. Spirit will guide you, but you must stay in touch with spirit for this to happen. The eternal self has to be nurtured into existence. In other words, if I don't do me, I don't get done. And *doing me* means simply self-creation.

Ah, self-creation. This is our human destiny—our true purpose in life. Creating one's self, or nurturing yourself into an existence you proudly love, can involve the smallest act of loving-kindness or the largest undertaking of detoxifying the world. It can entail an earthly experience or something of an entirely spiritual nature. As you nurture your soul, you allow air, touch, food, water, rest, sights, sounds, aromas, and movement to likewise nurture the physical layer of your existence. This is how we find and radiate synergy.

This blending of the health, fitness, and beauty arenas has a tremendous amount to do with the advancement of the Internet. Today, people communicate and seek out tremendous amounts of information with the click of a mouse. In the 1930s, the French scientist-priest Pierre Teilhard de Chardin predicted that there would be a shift from biological evolution to technological evolution and that God, through technology, would wrap the earth inside a "thinking skin." The Internet is this "thinking skin." Every one of you has the ability to experience the magic and mystery of this domain.

If you have never used a computer or gone online, don't let this faze you. Take a basic computer class or ask an Internet-savvy friend for help in exchange for a haircut, manicure, massage, or dinner. If you don't have a computer, go to a library and use theirs, or go to a local cyber café.

Once you feel comfortable behind the mouse, check out online communities. Behind The Chair at www.behindthechair.com is a great place to start. Another great community is www.modernsalon.com. My friend Teri Donnelly has an excellent site called The Cutting Club— www.cuttingclub.com. There are many others as well.

It is so important to connect with your community of like-minded individuals. This is a very important part of our wholeness—to feel connected to others.

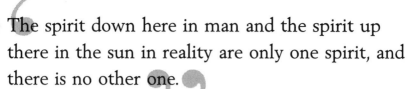

> **"**The spirit down here in man and the spirit up there in the sun in reality are only one spirit, and there is no other one.**"**
>
> *Upanishads*

Visit at least one beauty and/or wellness site on the Internet today. Make yourself a cup of organic tea and stay there for a while. Read several articles. Check out links. Join a chat session. Communicate with the site's administrators or webmaster if you have any pertinent questions or simply have comments.

Sites I enjoy or will soon check out:

_____

_____

_____

_____

_____

_____

_____

_____

Our True Self

Our spirit is floating fluidly and freely along the waves of another frequency domain—another energy field. This is the field of infinite possibilities. Spirit is spaceless, timeless, and eternal—it is the real you. Just as a radio captures Beethoven floating along the radio waves, through time and space, our central nervous system captures the real you—spirit—in your body and mind, so that you may experience your humanity within this existence. Depending on your level of consciousness, you will know this on a certain level. With our perceptions dulled, distracted, and busy attending to matters of the ego, communing with our higher selves takes some doing.

> Living in the present fuses the observer and the observed, harmonizing the mind. Once this is set in motion, the higher functions of evolution take over and start moving on their own account. Look at yourself with clear eyes and the rest will take care of itself.
>
> *Yatri*

Great Aspirations

We all have the power to raise our levels of consciousness from ordinary waking, sleeping, and dreaming states until we reach a level where we glimpse the soul. As we continue along the path to where we have such awareness, we move onto a higher level of consciousness. We begin to understand that spirit lives inside us. When achieving full enlightenment, we merge with spirit, and the whole universe becomes our body. As the ancient Vedic saying states—as is the atom, so is the universe; as is the microcosm, so is the macrocosm; as is the human body, so is the cosmic body; as is the human mind, so is the cosmic mind.

It is at this level of consciousness that we realize who we truly are. This level of enlightenment may take a lifetime—or many lifetimes. But you'll know it when you get there.

Continue to Explore

In this experiential journey that we've shared, you may have experienced an awakening of sorts. That's great, but remember, there's always more to learn. Keep asking your questions. Who am I? What am I here for? What are my gifts? Where did I come from? Are we alone in the universe? Why is there suffering? What can I do to be healed? Why is there evil? Who will love me? What is my path? How much is enough? In loving these questions and asking them over and over again, we remind ourselves that life is not a problem to be solved, but indeed a mystery to be explored. As Rainer Maria Rilke said, "Be patient toward all that is unsolved in your heart and try to love the questions themselves."

> *Go* confidently in the direction of your dreams.
> Live the life you've imagined. As you simplify
> your life, the laws of the universe will be simpler.*
>
> *Henry David Thoreau*

With an Open Heart

I continue to be moved so deeply by the members of our community. Beauty and wellness professionals are incredibly big-hearted—so open and loving—so intuitive and creative. These are our friends, our confidants, our peers, our guests. As an avid organic gardener, I liken our community to my backyard plot. Each season, I plant seeds. As life begins and continues to fruitfully grow, I tend to the weeding and watering. Finally, I harvest the delicious and nourishing bounty. With great thankfulness, I use the mature plants to nourish my body, decorate my home, heal my entire self. The energy and information from the plants become the energy and information of my mindbody physiology. How beautiful this is!

Tend to your inner garden. Plant the seeds of hope and dreams, relationships, and experiences; weed out the beliefs and emotions that hinder prolific and fruitful growth; and enjoy the delectable harvest. Know that your metaphoric garden, like your career, is an ongoing journey—holistic and cyclical—just like the rhythms of nature. This is the Cosmic Dance. So come on, grab a partner or kick up your heels solo, move your whole body of knowledge to the beat. Watch yourself getting into the rhythm. You *really* are beautiful!

Our deepest fear is not that we are inadequate.

Our deepest fear is that we are
powerful beyond measure. It is our light, not our
darkness, that most frightens us. We ask ourselves, who
am I to be brilliant, gorgeous, fabulous, talented?

Actually, who are you not to be?

You are a child of God. Your playing small does not serve the world. There is nothing enlightened about shrinking so that other people won't feel insecure around you. We were born to make manifest the glory of God that is within us. It is not in some of us; it is in everyone.

And as we let our light shine, we unconsciously give other people permission to do the same.

As we are liberated from our own fear, our presence automatically liberates others.

—*Nelson Mandela*

Notes:

Resources

Professional Education/Membership Organizations and Web Sites

The International Spa Association (ISPA): 859-226-4374, **www.experienceispa.com**

SpaElegance.Com: A premier e-marketplace for the Spa Industry. 877-200-SPAS, **www.SpaElegance.com**

The National Cosmetology Association: 312-527-6765, **www.salonprofessionals.org**

The Salon Association: 800-211-4TSA, **www.salons.org**

The International Nail Technicians Association (INTA): 312-321-5161, **www.IsNow.com**

Behind the Chair: For the cosmetologist and salon professional. 800-760-3010, **www.behindthechair.com**

Cosmetologists Chicago/Midwest Beauty Show: 312-321-6809, **www.IsNow.com**

Beautynet.com: The virtual salon for beauty, wellness, and style. 416-869-3131, **www.beautynet.com**

IB/Industrybuzz: Your source for industry news. **www.industrybuzz.net**

Rare NYC/Ruth Roche: Educational programs, tools, and inspiration. 212-253-6254, toll-free 866-RARENYC, **www.rarenyc.com**

The Cutting Club: Teri Donnelly's site. 877-CUT-CLUB, **www.cuttingclub.com**

The Christian Hairdressers Association: 847-419-8850, **www.christianhairdressers.com**

Club Salon: **www.clubsalon.com**

Stress Management and Health Enhancement Programs

The Chopra Center for Well Being. For multi-day programs, seminars, workshops, Chopra Center Services, or to locate a certified educator in your area (International network of educators who teach Chopra Center Seminars including: Primordial Sound Meditation, Creating Health, and Magical Beginnings—Enchanted Lives), call 888-424-6772 or 858-551-7788. Visit them at **www.chopra.com**. The Chopra Center is also a resource for Heartmath's software.

The Janssen Source, Inc.: 847-934-0923, **www.janssensource.com** or **MBJF@aol.com**. Programs include "Creating Health" as well as customized programs—with an emphasis on "wholeness in body, mind, and spirit" as well as beauty and wellness integration—to suit your specific needs, for companies large and small.

The Himalayan Institute—Center for Health and Healing. Rejuvenation Programs in a retreat setting. 570-253-5551, ext. 5000, **www.himalayaninstitute.org**

The Institute of Heartmath: 831-338-8500, **www.heartmath.org.** Through innovative research on positive emotions and physiology, Heartmath offers tools and techniques that improve learning, perfomance, and quality of life. Ask about their Freeze-Framer, an interactive software-based performance enhancement system that allows people to see and understand relationships between their heart rythms, emotions, mantal clarity, and performance. This would be an amazing offering in your holistic spa or for your salon/ spa staff.

Omega Institute for Holistic Studies: A retreat facility in Rhinebeck, New York, offering innovative workshops and retreats to rejuvenate the mind, body, and spirit with world-renowned faculty. 800-944-1001, **www.eomega.org**, ask for their catalog

Feathered Pipe Foundation. Located in Montana, top-notch yoga programs. 406-442-8196, **www.featheredpipe.com**

Association for Worksite Health Promotion. Ask about their membership, conferences, and quarterly publication, *Worksite Health*. 847-480-9574, **www.awhp.org**

National Wellness Institute. Membership provides a tremendous amount of benefits, resources, and their conference held each year is international in scope. 800-244-8922, **www.wellnessnwi.org/nwa/**

Wellness Councils of America: Membership, resources, conferences. 402-572-3590, **www.welcoa.org**. There are local affiliates around the country.

Wellness Councils of Canada: 800-263-2670

The National Health Observance Calendar is a great supplement planner for wellness programs at the worksite. Access at the National Wellness Institute and Wellness Councils Web sites or order a copy. Contact the National Health Information Center at 800-336-4797.

Integrative Medicine/Health Resources

The National Institute for Occupational Safety and Health (NIOSH) at the Centers for Disease Control and Prevention (CDC): Incredible information Service from EMF's in the workplace, to cancer, to AIDS, and the list goes on. 800-35-NIOSH, **www.cdc.gov/niosh/homepage.html**

American Holistic Health Association: A national resource connecting people with vital solutions for reaching a higher level of wellness. 714-779-6152, **www.ahha.org**

Center for Cancer Prevention at Harvard School of Public Health, Boston. The center's Web site helps individuals evaluate their risks of different types of cancer. **www.yourcancerrisk.harvard.edu**

American Botanical Council: A nonprofit that offers information on herbs and medicinal plants. 512-331-8868, **www.herbalgram.org**

Herb Research Foundation: A nonprofit that provides herbal therapy information. 800-748-2617, **www.herbs.org/herbs**

National Center for Homeopathy: A nonprofit membership organization that provides information on and practitioners of homeopathy. 703-548-7790, **www.healthy.net/nch**

American Academy of Medical Acupuncture: Basic information about acupuncture and referrals to M.D.s and osteopaths who practice acupuncture. 800-521-2262, **www.medicalacupuncture.org**

The American Dietetic Association: Referrals to dietitians in your area. You can also talk to a registered dietitian on the phone on various health-and-nutrition topics. 800-366-1655, **www.eatright.org**

American Chiropractic Association: General information on chiropractic care and practitioners in your area. 800-986-4636, **www.amerchiro.org/aca**

Academy for Guided Imagery: Trains health professionals on guided imagery. Materials available and referrals to practitioners in your area. 800-726-2070, **www.healthy.net/agi**

American Association of Naturopathic Physicians: Provides information about naturopathy, and referral to practitioners. 206-298-0126, **www.naturopathic.org**

American Academy of Dermatology: Information and resources for hair and skin. 888-462-DERM, **www.aad.com**

American Optometric Association: 888-396-3937, **www.aoanet.org**

To locate an optometrist specializing in vision therapy, contact the College of Optometrists in Vision Development (619-425-6191) or the Optometric Extension Program Foundation (714-250-8070).

U.S. Department of Health and Human Services: 202-619-0257, toll-free 877-696-6775, **www.healthfinder.gov**

The National Association for Holistic Aromatherapy: 888-ASK-NAHA, **www.naha.org**

HealthWorld Online: Wellness, self-care, fitness, nutrition and more. The most often visited natural health site on the Internet. **www.healthy.net**

The Massage Therapy Association: 847-864-0123, **www.amtamassage.org**. They also provide a locator service to find a practitioner near you.

Reflexology Association of America: **www.reflexology-usa.org**. Send inquiries to: Reflexology Association of America, 4012 Rainbow, Ste. K-PMB#585, Las Vegas, NV, 89103-2059.

Spa Finders: To find a destination or day spa near you. 800-ALL-SPAS, **www.spafinders.com**

Retreats International: Silence, serenity, and self-improvement retreats. 800-556-4532, **www.retreatsintl.org**

The U.S. National Library of Medicine: 301-594-5983, toll-free 888-FIND-NLM, **www.nlm.nih.gov**

American Heart Association: 800-AHA-USA1, **www.amhrt.org**

National Institutes of Health: **www.nih.gov**

Database at the National Institutes of Health: **www.odp.od.nih.gov/ods/databases/ibids.html**

OSHA—Occupational Safety and Health Administration/U.S. Dept of Labor: **www.OSHA.com**

The National Mental Health Association: 800-969-6642, **www.nmha.org**

The National Association for Mental Illness: 800-950-NAMI, **www.nami.org**

The Holistic Dental Association: Information and locating holistic dentists. 800-388-8124, **www.HolisticDental.org**

OneBody, Inc.: Source for professional practitioners in the healing arts. 888-646-5729, **www.onebody.com**

The Colour Energy Corporation: To find color therapy practitioners in your area or for more information. 604-687-3757, toll-free 800-225-1226, **www.colourenergy.com**

SAD (seasonal affective disorder): Information and light-therapy products. **www.lighttherapyproducts.com**

NSF International (National Sanitation Foundation): Get their NSF International Consumer Drinking Water book. 800-673-8010, **www.nsf.org**

Silver Lake Research: Watersafe drinking water test. 888-438-1942, **www.silverlakeresearch.com**

Feet First: Healthful information, products, shoes. 800-FEET-FIRST, **www.lauranormanreflexology.com**

Aromatherapy

National Association for Holistic Aromatherapy: 888-ASK-NAHA, **www.naha.org**

Environmental Medicine/Health

Dr. Makris is a nationally recognized expert on environmental impacts on human health and environmental diseases. 847-458-2596, **www.optimum healthmanagement.com** or **drmakris@earthlink.net**

Dr. Joseph Mercola's Optimal Wellness: One of the most visited natural health sites in the world (excellent nutrition information). This is my personal doctor. He has a specialty in environmental medicine. Sign up for his online newsletter. 847-985-1777, **www.mercola.com**

American Academy of Environmental Medicine. Focuses on illnesses caused by toxic or allergic reactions to environmental substances. Offers a referral service and literature. 913-642-6062, **www.healthy.net/aaem**

Rachel's Environment and Health News/Environmental Research Foundation: Understandable scientific information about human health and the environment. 888-272-2435, **www.rachel.org**

Environmental Working Group: Cutting edge research on health and the environment: Washington D.C. office, 202-667-6982, California office, 510-444-0973, **www.ewg.org**

Environmental Protection Agency: Wide range of health related issues. Ask for their Indoor Air Quality Product and Service Guide; they also have a safe water hotline. 800-426-4791, **www.epa.gov**

Seventh Generation: A leading producer of non-toxic cleaning products. Detailed information and resource links. 802-658-1771, **www.seventhgen.com**

Sound Health

Hearing protection for the workplace, anti-noise devices, sound cancellation technology:

Noise Suppression Technologies: 614-258-4455, **www.noisesuppression.com**
Conney Safety Products: 800-854-6860, **www.conney.com**
No Danger Electromagnetic Mobile Phone Shield for your cell phone: 888-256-2006

Sound Healers/Healing

Steven Halpern is an award-winning composer, recording artist, and sound healer—for over 25 years, a passionate advocate of the healing powers of music for health and spiritual growth. Music for everything from chakra balancing, to yoga, to meditation, massage, nature sound compositions, and more. 800-909-0707, **www.innerpeacemusic.com**, e-mail **innerpeace@innerpeacemusic.com**

Don Campbell is a trained classical magician, composer, and author of groundbreaking books on music and healing. For information on books by Don Campbell, or to order "Mozart Effect" recordings, contact: Mozart Effect Resource Center, 800-721-2177, **www.mozarteffect.com**

Nutrition

Tufts University Nutrition Navigator: Lists and rates more than 100 nutrition Web sites, **www.navigator.tufts.edu**

Local Harvest: Resource for finding food grown near your home, **www.localharvest.org**

Slow Food: An international movement celebrating the joy of eating. International office, 39 (0) 172 419611, U.S. office, 212-988-5146, **www.slowfood.com**

The Organic Consumers Association. Campaigning for food safety, organic agriculture, fair trade, and sustainability. 218-226-4164, **www.organicconsumers.org** and **www.purefood.org**

Organic Trade Association: Detailed information on organics, with many links. 413-774-7511, **www.ota.com**

The International Food Information Council Foundation: Publishes a variety of food safety and nutrition news; information on everything from vitamin E to mad cow disease. **http://ificinfo.health.org**

USDA Nutrient Data Laboratory: USDA's food composition database. **www.nal.usda.gov/fnic/foodcomp**

Ergonomics

Direct Safety Company: Ergonomically sound health and safety products/furniture for the beauty professional. 800-528-7405 or 602-968-7009 for catalog, **www.directsafety.com**

The American Academy of Orthopedic Surgeons: Offers a comprehensive brochure, "Lift It Safe," on how to avoid back pain. 800-824-2663, **www.aos.org**

"Health and Safety for Hair Care and Beauty Professionals," from the Labor Occupational Health Program at the University of California at Berkeley: A teaching curriculum on work hazards that includes detailed information on ergonomic problems and their solutions. 510-642-5507

Mindfulness in Motion and Fitness

Health and Fitness Information and Online Coaching and Personal Training:

Asimba, Inc.: 650-367-1800, **www.asimba.com**

GymAmerica.com: **www.gymamerica.com**

Fitness Zone: 205-324-1955 or 800-875-9145, **www.fitnesszone.com**

FitnessLink: 908-689-8725, **www.fitnesslink.com**

IDEA Health and Fitness Association: 800-999-4332, **www.ideafit.com**

National Association of Governor's Councils on Physical Fitness and Sports: **www.fitnesslink.com/Govcouncil/**

ACE, American Council on Exercise: 800-529-8227, **acefitness.org**

The Pilates Center: Information and finding a certified instructor in your area. 800-474-5283, **pilatesstudio.com**

The American Society for the Alexander Technique: 800-473-0620, **www.alexandertech.org**

American Dance Therapy Association: Dance/movement therapies. 410-997-4048, **www.adta.org**

Rubenfeld Synergy Method: In the United States, the National Association of Rubenfeld Synergists, 877-RSM-2468; in Canada, the Canadian Association of Rubenfeld Synergists, 519-669-8427; **www.rubenfeldsynergy.com**

Trance Dance: The Natale Institute, 512-708-8888, **www.trancedance.com**

Hand Health Unlimited: Products and programs for helping hands work and feel better. 513-868-7933 or 888-868-HAND, **www.handhealth.com**

Yoga

The Yoga Site: A premier online yoga resource for all things yoga—teachers, retreats, education, supplies, etc. **yogasite.com**

Yoga Zone: 800-264-9642, **www.yogazone.com**

YogaPro: 800-488-8414, **www.yogapro.com**

Yoga Journal: 800-436-9642, **www.yogajournal.com**

Yoga International Magazine: Published by the Himalayan International Institute, a nonprofit organization; for subscriptions, 800-229-6243, **www.HimalayanInstitute.org**

Extense yoga programs/videos for the beauty professional: Christopheray, 877-EXTENSE, e-mail **christopheray@msn.com**

Humor Resources

The Humor Project, Inc.: 518-587-8770, **www.humorproject.com**
Jest for the Health of It!: 831-475-9570, **www.jesthealth.com**
L.A.U.G.H.S.—Laughing At and Understanding Good Humor Seminars:
617-288-8664, **www.laughsrus.com**
Humor Heals: 773-PLACEBO, **www.humorheals.com**
American Association for Therapeutic Laughter (AATH): 602-995-1454,
www.aath.org

Positive Affirmations

Louise Hay at Hay House: Books, audios, videos and other products. Metaphysical teacher and best-selling author, Hay has assisted thousands discover and use full potential of their own creative powers for personal growth and self-healing. 800-654-5126, **www.hayhouse.com**

Holistic and Organic Companies (Web sites and catalogs): From water and air purification systems to organic body care, cleaning products and clothing, to programs for learning color therapy, yoga, vision improvement, toning, full spectrum lighting . . . and the list goes on.

New Life Systems: Premier full-service professional supplier of products for the salon, spa, and massage industries. 800-852-3082, **www.newlifesystems.com**

Serenity: Music to Awaken the Heart: 800-869-1684, **serenity@bright.net**, **www.serenitymusic.com**

Natural Lifestyle Suppliers: 800-752-2775

Healthyeverything.com: A wide variety of natural and chemical-free products, this site has beautiful organic clothing. 800-887-6901, **www.healthyeverything.com**

Alternatives for Simple Living: 712-274-8875, **www.simpleliving.org**

Lifekind Products: Wide variety of organic and naturally safer products. 800-284-4983, **www.lifekind.com**

Gaiam "Conscience Commerce": A wide variety of lifestyle items for living simply, organically, and naturally. This site includes the Harmony, Real Goods, Self-Care, and Living Arts companies. Call at their individual phone numbers: Harmony, 800-869-3446; Self Care, 800-345-3371; Real Goods (products for an ecologically sustainable future), 800-762-7325; Living Arts (great source for yoga education, clothing, props, etc., as well as practices and products for total well-being), 800-254-8464. Access all at **www.gaiam.com**.

As We Change: A marketplace for women. From Reflexology clogs to natural lubricants to nourishing skin and hair care products, this site addresses a variety of feminine concerns as well as practices and products for enhancing vitality and reducing stress. 800-203-5585, **www.aswechange.com**

WholeLife: A resource for natural health, personal development, and sustainable living, with an emphasis on a holistic approach to beauty and well-being. They conduct conferences as well as market a wide variety of natural and organic products. 800-551-3976, **www.wholelife.com**

Sounds True: Audio and video for the inner life. 800-333-9185, **www.soundstrue.com**

Lab Safety Supply: Ventilation systems and referrals to certified industrial hygienists. 800-356-0783, **www.labsafety.com**

Light Energy Company: Full spectrum lights for the home and workplace. 800-544-4826

Quantum Pure Air Corporation: A source for ozone purification systems. 401-732-6770

Technology Alternatives Corporation: Source for gaussmeters to measure EMFs (electromagnetic frequencies). 800-638-9121, **www.milligauss.com**

Online Spiritual Communities/Web Sites

BeliefNet, Inc.: A multifaith ecommunity. **www.Beliefnet.com**

AmericanCatholic.org: 513-241-5615, **www.americancatholic.org**

Virtual Jerusalem: Excellent resource for Judaism. **www.virtualjerusalem.com**

IslamiCity: Global Muslim ecommunity. 310-642-0006, **www.Islamicity.org**

HinduNet, Inc.: 617-698-1106, **www.hindunet.org**

DharmaNet International: Gateways to Buddhism. **www.dharmanet.org**

The Christian Hairdressers Association: 847-419-8850, **www.christianhairdressers.com**

The Chopra Center for Well Being: 888-4CHOPRA (424-6772), **www.chopra.com**

A portion of the proceeds from the sale of this book will go toward the Xenon Foundation:

"The Xenon Foundation"
Please open your hearts and help us make Xenon's wish come true. The Foundation's cause is two-fold. It can let others live the dream of becoming a beauty professional through The Xenon Foundation Scholarship Program. It also can help in financially assisting fellow beauty professionals stricken with a catastrophic disease.

To receive information or to contribute to the Xenon Foundation, contact Janice McCafferty:

Phone: (773) 736-9034
Fax: (773) 202-8074
e-mail: **XenonFoundation@aol.com**

Bibliography and Recommended Reading

Spirituality and Philosophy

The American Paradox: Spiritual Hunger in an Age of Plenty. David G. Myers. Yale University Press, 2001.

The Aquarian Conspiracy. Marilyn Ferguson. J.P. Tarcher, Inc., 1980.

Bhagavad-Gita. Any one of the over 200 translations that resonates with you.

The Bible. Any issue that resonates with you.

Changing for Good. James O Prochaska, John C. Norcross, Carlos C. Diclemente. Avon, 1995.

The Coming of the Cosmic Christ. Matthew Fox. Harper & Row, 1998.

A Course in Miracles. Viking Press, 1996.

Don't Sweat the Small Stuff—and It's All Small Stuff. Richard Carlson. Hyperion, 1997.

The Dream of the Earth. Thomas Berry. Sierra Club Books, 1988.

The Experience Economy: Work Is Theater and Every Business a Stage. Joseph Pine & James H. Gilmore. Harvard Business School Publishing, 1999.

The Four Agreements: A Practical Guide to Personal Freedom. Don Miguel Ruiz. Amber Allen Publishing, 1997.

Future Shock. Alvin Toffler. Bantam Books, 1991.

How to Know God. Deepak Chopra, M.D. Harmony Books, 2000.

On Caring. Milton Meyeroff. Harperperrenial Library, 1990.

An Open Heart: Practicing Compassion in Everyday Life. The Dalai Lama. Little, Brown and Company, 2001.

Original Blessing. Matthew Fox. Bear & Co., 1983.

The Path of Love. Deepak Chopra, M.D. Harmony, 1997.

Peace in Every Step: The Path of Mindfulness in Everyday Life. Thich Nhat Hanh. Bantam Books, 1992.

Restoring the Earth. Kenny Ausubel, H. J. Kramer. 1997.

Rituals for Sacred Living. Jane Alexander. New York: Sterling Publishing Co., Inc., 1999.

The Seven Spiritual Laws of Success. Deepak Chopra, M.D. New World Library, 1994.

The Spirit of Place: A Workbook of Sacred Alignment: Ceremonies and Visualizations for Cultivating Your Relationship with the Earth. Loreen Cruden. Destiny Books, 1995.

A Spirituality Named Compassion. Matthew Fox. HarperCollins, 1990.

The Soul of the Firm. William Pollard. Zondervan Publishing House, 2000.

Taking the Fear Out of Changing. Dennis O'Grady. Adams Media Corporation, 1993.

Voluntary Simplicity: Toward a Way of Life That Is Outwardly Simple, Inwardly Rich. Duane Elgin. Quill/William Morrow, 1993.

Waking Up in Time. Peter Russell. Origin Press, 1998.

The Way of the Shaman. Michael Harner, Ph.D. HarperCollins, 1990.

The Web of Life. Fritjof Capra. An Anchor Book, 1996.

Who Moved My Cheese? An Amazing Way to Deal with Change in Your Work and in Your Life. Spencer Johnson, Kenneth H. Blanchard. Putnam Publishing Group, 1998.

Working from the Heart. Jacqueline McMakin with Sonya Dyer. HarperCollins, 1993.

Mindbody Health/Healing

Ageless Body, Timeless Mind. Deepak Chopra, M.D. Harmony Books, 1993.

The Art of Reflexology. Inge Dougans with Suzanne Ellis. Barnes and Noble Books, 1995.

Ayurveda: Secrets of Healing. Maya Tiwari. Lotus Press, 1995.

Ayurveda: The Science of Self Healing. Dr. Vasant Lad. Lotus Press, 1984.

Body, Mind, and Sport. John Douillard. D.C., Crown Publishing, 1994.

The Complete Guide to Natural Healing. Tom Monte and the Editors of *Natural Health Magazine.* Perigree Books, 1997.

Creative Visualization. Shakti Gawain. Bantam Books, 1985.

Divine Intuition. Lynn A Robinson, M.Ed. Dorling Kindersley, 2001.

Encyclopedia of Natural Medicine. Michael Murray, N.D., and Joseph Pizzorno, N.D. Prima Publishing, 1991.

Flower Essence Repertory: A Comprehensive Guide to North American and English Flower Essences for Emotional and Spiritual Well-Being. Patricia Kaminski and Richard Katz. Published by the Flower Essence Society; contact at 800-548-0075.

The Living Beauty Detox Program. Ann Louise Gittleman, M.S., C.N.S. Harper-Collins, 2000.

The Nature Doctor. H.C.A. Vogel. Instant Improvement, Inc., 1991.

Perfect Health. Deepak Chopra, M.D. Harmony, 1991.

Radical Healing: Integrating the World's Great Therapeutic Traditions to Create a Transformative Medicine. Rudolph Ballentine, M.D. Harmony Books, 1999.

Reiki Fire. Frank Arjava Petter. Lotus Light/Shangri-La, 2000.

The Relaxation Response. Herbert Benson, M.D. Wholecare, 2000.

Spontaneous Healing. Andrew Weil, M.D. Knopf, 1995.

Trance Dance: The Dance of Life. Frank Natale. Element, 1995.

Vibrational Medicine: New Choices for Healing Ourselves. Richard Gerber, M.D. Bear & Co., 1988.

Wheels of Life: A User's Guide to the Chakra System. Anodea Judith. Llewellyn Publications, 1987.

Wheels of Light: Chakras, Auras, and the Healing Energy of the Body. Rosalyn L. Bruyere. A Fireside Book, 1994.

Wherever You Go, There You Are: Mindfulness Meditation in Everyday Life. Jon Kabat-Zinn. Hyperion, 1994.

The Wisdom of Healing. David Simon, M.D. Harmony Books, 1997.

Women's Bodies, Women's Wisdom. Christiane Northrup, M.D. Bantam, 1994.

The Women's Complete Healthbook. The American Medical Women's Association. Delacorte Press, 1995.

You Can Feel Good Again: Common-Sense Therapy for Releasing Depression and Changing Your Life. Richard Carlson. Plume, 1994.

Environmental Health

Chemical Exposures—Low Levels and High Stakes. Nicholas A. Ashford and Claudia S. Miller. Van Nostrand Reinhold, 1991.

The Consumer's Guide to Effective Environmental Choices: Practical Advice from the Union of Concerned Scientists. Michael Brower Ph.D and Warren Leon, Ph.D, Three Rivers Press, 1999.

Electromagnetic Fields: What You Need to Know to Protect Your Health. Laurie Tarkan. Bantam Books, 1994.

Feng Shui Handbook: How to Create a Healthier Living and Working Environment. Master Lam Kam Chuen. Henry Holt and Co., Inc., 1996.

How to Grow Fresh Air: Fifty Houseplants That Purify Your Home and Office. B.C. Wolverton. Penguin Books, 1997.

The Ion Effect: How Air Electricity Rules Your Life and Health. Fred Soyka with Alan Edmonds. Bantam Books, 1977.

Light: Medicine of the Future. Jacob Liberman. Bear & Co., 1991.

Living Healthy in a Toxic World. David Steinman and R. Michael Wisner. Berkley Publishing, 1996.

The Nontoxic Home & Office: Protecting Yourself and Your Family from Everyday Toxics and Health Hazards. Debra Lynn Dadd. G.P. Putnam's Sons, 1992.

Pandora's Poison: Chlorine, Health, and a New Environmental Strategy. Joe Thornton. MIT, 2000.

The Poisoning of Our Homes and Workplaces. Jack Thrasher, Ph.D., and Alan Broughton M.D. Seadora, Inc., 1989.

Sacred Space: Clearing and Enhancing the Energy of Your Home. Denise Linn. Ballantine, 1995.

The Safe Shopper's Bible: A Consumer's Guide to Nontoxic Household Products, Cosmetics, and Food. David Steinman and Samuel Epstein, M.D. Macmillan, 1995.

Spiritual Housecleaning: Healing the Space Within by Beautifying the Space Around You. Kathryn Robyn. New Harbinger Publications.

Warning: The Electricity Around You May Be Hazardous to Your Health. Ellen Sugarman. Simon & Shuster, New York, 1992.

You Are What You Breathe. Robert Massy. University of the Trees Press, 1980.

Vision Therapy

The Eye Care Revolution. Robert Abel Jr., M.D. Kensington Publishing Corporation, 1999.

Natural Eye Care: An Encyclopedia. Mark Grossman, O.D., L.Ac., and Glen Swartwout, O.D. Kent Publishing, 1999; also **www.visionworkusa.com** or call 888-735-8475.

Seven Steps to Better Vision. Richard Leviton. 1992.

Sensory Awareness/Modulation

The Art of Calm: Relaxation Through the Five Senses. Brian Luke Seaward, Ph.D. Health Communications, Inc., 1999.

A Natural History of the Senses. Diane Ackerman. Vintage, 1990.

Sensuous Living. Nancy Conger. Llewellyn Publications, 1995.

The Spell of the Sensuous. David Abram. Vintage Books, 1996.

Sound and Music

The Healing Voice: Traditional & Contemporary Toning, Chanting & Singing. Joy Gardner-Gordon. Crossing Press, 1993.

The Mozart Effect. Don Campbell. Avon Books, 1997.

Music: Physician for Times to Come. Don Campbell. Quest Books, 1991.

Sounds of Healing. Mitchell Gaynor, M.D. Avon Books, 1999.

Nutrition and Herbal Therapy

Aphrodite: A Memoir of the Senses. Isabel Allende. HarperPerennial, 1998.

Diet for Natural Beauty: A Natural Anti-Aging Formula for Skin and Hair. Aveline Kushi with Wendy Esko and Maya Tiwari. Japan Publications, Inc., 1991.

Earl Mindell's Food as Medicine. Earl Mindell. Fireside, 1994.

Earl Mindell's Herb Bible. Earl Mindell, R. Ph., Ph.D. Fireside, 1992.

Earl Mindell's Supplement Bible. Earl Mindell. Fireside, 1998.

Earl Mindell's Vitamin Bible for the 21st Century. Earl Mindell. Warner Books, 1999.

Eat, Drink, and Be Healthy. Walter C. Willett, M.D. Free Press/Simon & Schuster, Inc., 2001.

Eating Well for Optimum Health. Andrew Weil, M.D. Quill, 2001.

Eating with Conscience: The Bioethics of Food. D. Michael W. Fox. NewSage Press, 1997.

Feeding the Body: Nourishing the Soul. Deborah Kesten, M.P.H. Conari Press, 1997.

The Food Doctor: Healing Foods for Mind and Body. Vicki Edgson Dipion and Ian Marber Dipion. Collins & Brown Ltd., 1999.

The Healing Secrets of Food. Deborah Kesten, M.P.H. New World Library, 2001.

Herbs for Health and Happiness. Mo Siegal and Nancy Burke. Time Life Books, 1999.

The New Holistic Herbal. David Hoffman. Element, 1990.

Nourishing Traditions: The Cookbook That Challenges Politically Correct Nutrition and the Diet Dictocrats, 2nd edition. Sally Fallon with Mary G. Enig, Ph.D. New Trends Publishing, Inc., 1999.

Prescription for Nutritional Healing, 3rd edition. James F. Balch, M.D., and Phyllis A. Balch, C.N.C. Avery/A Member of Penguin Putnam Inc., 1997.

Why Weight: A Guide to End Compulsive Eating. Geneen Roth. Penguin, 1989.

Color Therapy

The Color Therapy Workbook: A Guide to the Use of Color for Health and Healing. Theo Gimbel. Element, 1993.

Discover the Magic of Color. Lillian Verner Bonds. Optima, 1993.

The Miracle of Color Healing. Vicky Wall. The Aquarian Press, 1993.

General Beauty and Wellness

Aveda Rituals. Horst Rechelbacher. Henry Holt and Company, LLC, 1999.

A Consumers Dictionary of Cosmetic Ingredients, 5th edition. Ruth Winter, M.S. Three Rivers Press, 1999.

Health Risks in Today's Cosmetics. Nicholas J Smeh. Alliance Publishing Company, 1994.

The Herbal Body Book. Stephanie Tourles. Storey Books, 1994.

Natural Foot Care. Stephanie Tourles. Storey Books, 1998.

Natural Hand Care. Norma Weinberg. Storey Books, 1998.

Natural Organic Hair and Skin Care. Aubrey Hampton. Organica Press, 1987.

Naturally Healthy Hair. Mary Beth Janssen. Storey Books, 1999.

Naturally Healthy Skin. Stephanie Tourles. Storey Books, 1999.

Radiant Beauty: Your Healthy and Organic Guide to Total Body Well-Being. Mary Beth Janssen. Rodale Press, 2001.

Ayurvedic Beauty and Wellness

Absolute Beauty: Radiant Skin and Inner Harmony Through the Ancient Secrets of Ayurveda. Pratima Raichur with Marion Cohn. HarperCollins, 1997.

Ayurvedic Beauty Care. Melanie Sachs. Lotus Press, 1994.

Yoga and Breathwork

The Healing Path of Yoga: Alleviate Stress, Open Your Heart, and Enrich Your Life. Nischala Joy Devi. Three Rivers Press, 2000.

Living Your Yoga: Finding the Spiritual in Everyday Life. Judith Lasater, Ph.D., P.T. Rodmell Press, 2000.

Mudras: Yoga in Your Hands. Gertrud Hirschi. Samuel Weiser, Inc., 2000.

Science of Breath. Swami Rama, Rudolph Ballentine, M.D., and Alan Hymes, M.D. The Himalayan Institute of Yoga Science and Philosophy, 1981.

Yoga: Mastering the Basics. Sandra Anderson and Rolf Sovik. Himalayan Institute Press, 2000.

Yoga, Mind & Body. Sivananda Yoga Vedanta Center. Dorling Kindersley, 1996.

Aromatherapy

The Aromatherapy Workbook. Marcel Lavabre. Healing Arts Press, 1990.

The Complete Book of Essential Oils and Aromatherapy. Valerie Ann Worwood. New World Library, 1991.

Magical Aromatherapy: The Power of Scent. Scott Cunningham. Llewellyn Publications, 1993.

The Practice of Aromatherapy. Jean Valnet M.D. Beekman Publishing, 1990.

Published Works/Education Specific to the Beauty Profession

Health Hazard Manual for Cosmetologists—Hairdressers, Beauticians, and Barbers. Nellie J. Brown, M.S., from Cornell University Chemical Hazard Information Program, published by New York State Department of Health/Bureau of Occupational Health, for single copies call 716-852-4191.

Milady Publishing Corporation: A wide range of continuing education programs— in seminar, workshop, book, and technology formats— for the beauty professional. Also, materials for the cosmetology school and educator. Call for further information, 800-223-8055, **www.milady.com**.

A Miracle in My Hands: A Stylist's Inspiration (and anything else published) by Douglas A. Cox. Contact at 800-789-9617 at extension 667.

Passion: A Salon Professional's Handbook for Building a Successful Business. Susie Fields Carder. Carder Creative Enterprises, 1995.

Pivot Point International: A wide range of continuing education programs—in seminar, workshop, book, and technology formats—for the beauty professional. Also, materials for the cosmetology school and educator. Call for further information, 800-886-HAIR, **www.pivot-point.com**.

Magazines/Web Sites

Professional Beauty Magazines/Web Sites in the United States

Advanstar Communications is the publisher of *American Salon* magazine (**www .americansalonmag.com**) and *American Spa* magazine (**www.americanspamag .com**). Subscribe to *American Salon* at **https://www.advanstar.com/subscribe/as** and to *American Spa* at **https://www.advanstar.com/subscribe/aspa**. Or call 1-800-598-6008 for more information.

Creative Age is the publisher of *Nailpro* (**www.nailpro.com**), *DAYSPA*® (**www.dayspa mag.com**), and *Professional Cosmetics*. For information call 800-442-5667.

Hair Color & Design. For subscription information contact 856-933-0111, ext. 204.

Salon News. For subscription information call 800-477-6411, **www.salonnews.com**

Vance Publishing is the publisher of *Modern Salon, Salon Today,* and *Process (Hair Color)* magazines. For subscription information call 847-634-2600, ext. 305; also go to **www.modernsalon.com**

Professional Beauty Magazines in Canada

The Canadian Hairdresser Magazine (published by Harco). 416-923-1111, **info@canhair.com**

Salon Magazine (published by Salon Communications, Inc.). 905-430-9723, **www.beautynet.com**

Professional Newsletter

TRENDzine!: An e-mail newsletter created by Jody Byrne that forecasts trends for the salon, spa, beauty, fashion, and wellness industries. To subscribe for your-self or a friend, send an e-mail to **TRENDzine@aol.com** and write subscribe in the subject line. You may also reach Jody Byrne, President of Trends and Sources International, at 330-626-3235.

Sprituality, Beauty, and Health Magazines

Healing Retreats and Spas: 805-962-7107, **www.healingretreats.com**

Natural Health: 800-526-8440, **www.naturalhealthmag.com**

New Age: The Journal for Holistic Living: 740-375-2332, **www.newage.com**

Organic Style: 800-365-3276, **www.organicstyle.com**

Personal Transformation: fax 918-683-2466, **www.personaltransformation.com**

Spa Finder Magazine: 800-ALL-SPAS, **www.spafinder.com**

"Spirit at Work": A wonderful newsletter that helps bring spiritual practices into the workplace. Call 203-467-9084 for a sample copy.

Spirituality and Health: 800-876-8202, **www.spiritualityhealth.com**

Index

Academy of Sciences and Sofia Medical
    Institute (Bulgaria), 196
acupuncture, 48–49
aerobic exercise, 107
affirmation. *See* positive affirmation
Air dosha, 56–59, 109, 158–161. *See
    also* Ayurveda
air quality, 75, 179–180
alcohol consumption, 152
Alexander Technique, 116
Allens, Hugh, 100
altars, 93
alternate-nostril breathing, 83–84
American Council on Exercise, 109
American Heart Association, 87, 138
American Massage Therapy Association,
    173–174
anorexia, 135
anti-noise technology, 203–204
antioxidants, 146
arm against wall stretch, 128
aromatherapy, 48–49, 181–184
asanas (postures), 111, 113. *See also*
    yoga
astringent taste, 160
Ayurveda, 53–57
    color therapy in, 193
    energy assessment, 58–61
    essential oils and, 184
    exercise and, 109
    mindbody principles of, 56–59
    nutrition and, 158–161
    vision and, 186

backbend stretch, 130
basal metabolic rate (MBR), 107

Base Chakra, 49
beauty
    attitude toward, 43–44
    exercise and, 98–99
    perception of, 189–190
    as spiritual entity, 41–43
beauty products
    chemicals in, 74–76
    flower essences as, 53
beauty services, 207–209. *See also* salons
    integrated with wellness, 44–46,
        48–49
    referrals to medical professionals,
        208
    sense of touch and, 171
    spirituality within, 30–31
Behind the Chair, 219
bicycling, 108
bitter taste, 160
blues, 199
Blues music, 199
Booth, Frank W., 100
bowing forward stretch, 127
breathing exercises, 80–81
    diaphragmatic, 81–83
    Pranayama techniques, 71, 83–86
    for yoga, 91–92, 112, 113
Brow Chakra, 50
bursitis, 121

Calypso music, 199
cancer, 146
carbohydrates, 140–141
carpal tunnel syndrome, 120
cat's pose, 131
cell phones, 204

Center for Neuroimmunology (Loma Linda University), 200
Centers for Disease Control (CDC), 142, 164–165
chairs, 125
chakra system, 49–51, 191–193
change, fear of, 10–12
chanting, 202
chemicals, 74–76, 173, 179–180. See also organic plants
child's pose, 131–132
Chinese medicine, 187
Chi-ung, 117
chlorine, 142
cholesterol, 107, 147–148
Chopra, Deepak, 88
Chopra Center for Well Being, 58, 90
chromatherapy, 191–193
cilia, 177
"clean" food, 136. See also nutrition
clients, 51–52, 209–211. See also beauty services; salons
color, 191–193
communication, 195
compassion, 36–37
conflict resolution, 35–36
consciousness, 220–221. See also meditation
Consumer Dictionary of Cosmetic Ingredients, A (Winter), 75
cortisol, 45, 173, 188
Course in Miracles, A (Foundation for Inner Peace), 79
creative visualization, 18–20
Crown Chakra, 50, 193
cumulative trauma disorders (CTDs), 120
Cutting Club, 219

dance, 114–116, 198
dehydration, 131. See also water
dental health, 164–165, 180, 205
depression, 188
detoxification, 173, 187
Devries, Stephen, 147
dharma, 15–16
dietary supplements. See vitamins
digestion process, 177–178
discs, herniated, 121
distress. See stress
Dixieland music, 199

Donnelly, Teri, 219
doshas, 56–59, 109, 158–161. See also Ayurveda
drumming circles, 199–200

ears, 204
Earth dosha, 56–59, 109, 158–161. See also Ayurveda
ear to shoulder stretches, 127
Eat, Drink, and Be Healthy (Willet), 149
eating disorders, 135
Einstein, Albert, 69
elbow pull, 128
electrical chairs, 125
electromagnetic frequencies (EMFs), 76
elimination, 66
emotions
    clearing processes for, 34–36, 65
    stress from, 69–70
endorphins, 103
energy
    Ayurveda questionnaire, 58–59
    balancing, 60–61
    chakra system, 49–51, 191–193
    life-force, 10–11
    nutrition and, 164
Environmental Defense Fund, 142
Environmental Working Group (EWG), 142
equipment, for salons, 124–125
ergonomics, 119–125
essential oils, 182. See also aromatherapy
    aromatherapy vs., 52
    Ayurveda and, 184
eustress, 71
exercise
    beauty and, 98–99
    benefits of, 96–98, 152
    chronic pain and, 120–121
    developing regimen for, 109–110, 112
    motivation for, 100–105
    preventing injuries during, 119–125
    setting goals for, 98, 106
    types of, 107–108, 114–118
eye care, 186–187

facialists' chairs, 125
fascia, 97
fast food, 138
fat, in diet, 140–141, 150
fears, 10–12

Feldenkrais Method, 116–117
fiber, 138
financial success, 20–22, 28–29
Fire dosha, 56–59, 109, 158–161. *See also* Ayurveda
flower essence therapy, 48–49, 52–53
Folan, Lilias, 114
food. *See* nutrition
Food Guide Pyramid, 148–151
forgiveness, 37
free radicals, 71–72
fruits, 151
fulfillment, 29
full-spectrum lighting, 188
Future Shock (Toffler), 68

gardening, 93
Great Chain of Being, 3
Gregorian Chant, 199
guided imagery. *See* creative visualization

hand and wrist poses, 123, 129
hands-clasped stretches, 128
Hara Chakra, 50, 192
head side to side stretch, 127
Healing Works Laugh Club, 23
health. *See also* health; *individual names of health conditions*
  benefits of Ayurveda, 53–54
  chronic pain and, 120–121
  dehydration, 141
  exercise and, 99–100
  Health Risk Appraisal (HRA), 76
  optimism and, 44–46
  wellness quotient, 47–48
Healthy Eating Pyramid, 149
heart. *See also* health
  breathing technique for, 14–15
  cholesterol guidelines, 147–148
  electromagnetic field of, 13
  exercise for, 106, 107
  meditation and, 87
  yoga for, 111
Heart Chakra, 50, 192
Hellerwork, 117
Heraclitis, 10
herbal drinks, 164
herniated discs, 121
Hierarchy of Needs theory, 28–29
Hindu culture
  chakra system, 49–51

Vedas, 88, 194, 221
  yoga in, 111
Holmes, Oliver Wendell, 211
homeostasis, 47
hormones
  cortisol, 45, 173, 188
  melatonin, 188
Houlihan, Jane, 142
How to Grow Fresh Air (Wolverton), 75
hydraulic chairs, 125
hygiene, personal, 180, 205

immune system, 44–45, 102
India, 53. *See also* Hindu culture
industrial safety, 75, 76
Institute of HeartMath, 13–14
interconnectedness, 216
International Association of Fitness Professionals (IDEA), 109
Internet, 218–220

Janssen, Mary Beth, 176
Jazz, 199
journal keeping, 12, 93
Journal of the American Medical Association (JAMA), 106

Kapalabhati breath, 85
Kapha dosha, 56–59. *See also* Ayurveda

laughing clubs, 23
lighting, 76, 119, 187–188
Lilias! (video), 114
Linn, Denise, 179
listening skills, 195
liver, 187
Living Arts videos, 114
Loma Linda University School of Medicine, 200

manicure tables, 125
mantra, 88, 202
Maslow, Abraham, 28–29
massage, 48–49, 66
  acquiring skills for, 175
  mindbody physiology and, 172–173
  preventing injuries while performing, 124
  self-care and, 173–177
  sense of touch, 169–172
  types of, 174–175

Material Safety Data Sheets (MSDS), 75

Mayo Clinic, 45

meditation, 48–49, 86–92. *See also* breathing exercises
exercise and, 108
mantra for, 88
nutrition and, 162
sounds for, 202

melatonin, 188

mentoring, 31–34

Michigan State University, 196

milk thistle, 187

mindbody physiology, 5, 46–47
Ayurveda and, 53–61
massage and, 172–173
optimism and, 44–46

Mind-Body Wellness Center, 200

mindfulness, 55–56. *See also* exercise

mind vs. brain, 168

modified shoulder stand, 126–127

monounsaturated fats, 140–141

Multiple Chemical Sensitivities Disorder, 74

music. *See also* sound
biochemical effects of, 197–199
drumming circles, 199–200
singing, 201
styles of, 199
as therapy, 196–197

Myofacial Release, 97

nadi shodhana, 83–84

Natale Institute, 115

National Institute of Environmental Health Sciences, 76

National Institutes of Health, 111

Native American culture
shamanism, 18–19, 199–200
smudging, 65

nature, Ayurveda and, 57

Navel Chakra, 50, 192

neck stretches, 127

needs, theory of, 28–29

negative ion environments, 179

Noëlle Spa for Beauty and Wellness, 90

"non-ordinary reality," 199–200

nutraceuticals, 145–147

nutrition, 65–66, 76, 164–165
Ayurveda and, 158–161
cholesterol guidelines, 147–148

"clean" food, 136
counseling in, 48–49, 137
for ear health, 204
eating habits, 136–139
for eye health, 187
fats, 140–141, 150
food and spirituality, 134–135, 155–158
food preparation, 158
grains, 150–151
guidelines for, 144–145, 148–151
meal planning, 152–154
nutrients, 140–141
organic food, 72–73, 136–137, 146
proteins, 140–141, 151
sense of smell and, 177–178
stress and, 162–163
vitamin sources, 146–147
Zone principle, 143

obesity, 135, 152

Occupational Safety and Health Administration (OSHA), 75, 76

Ohashiatsu, 117

Oldways Preservation and Exchange Trust, 149–150

"Om," 202

optimism, 44–46

organic plants, 72–73, 136–137, 146

Oriental healing arts, 174

Ortho-Bionomy, 117

overhead stretch, 128

palm stretches, 129–130

Passage, Leo, 20

physical activity. *See* exercise

physical needs, 28–29

phytonutrients, 145–147

Pilates, 117

pinched nerves, 121

Pitta dosha, 56–59. *See also* Ayurveda

polyunsaturated fats, 140–141

positive affirmation, 6–7, 10–16, 24
career choice and, 8–9, 17–18
child within and, 22–23
creative visualization and, 18–20
exercise and, 118
prosperity consciousness and, 20–22
for stress, 77

posture, 123. *See also* yoga

Prana, 83

Pranayama, 71, 83–86, 112, 113
prayer pose, 129
present-moment awareness, 17–18
prosperity, 20–22
proteins, 140–141, 151
pungent taste, 160

Qi Gong, 117

Radiant Beauty: Your Healthy and Organic Guide to Total Body Well-Being (Janssen), 176
Reflexology, 174
Reggae music, 199
Reiki, 52
research studies
    on chlorine, 142
    on dental health, 164–165
    on drumming, 200
    on meditation, 87
    on sound, 196–197
resiliency, 45
rest, 66, 177
Rilke, Maria, 221
rituals, 93
Rock and Roll music, 199
rolfing, 97
Romantic music, 199
Root Chakra, 49, 192
Rosen Method, 117
routine, importance of, 66
Rubenfield, Ilana, 118
Rubenfield Synergy Method, 118
running, 108
ruptured discs, 121

Sacred music, 199
Sacred Space (Linn), 179
safety
    during exercise, 119–120
    industrial, 75, 76
salons. *See also* beauty services
    chemicals in, 74–76
    Earth-friendly practices of, 72
    environment of, 61, 73–74
    equipment for, 124–125
    meditation space in, 90
    spirituality in, 61–63
    water availability in, 142
salty taste, 159–160
sanitation, in workplace, 76

Satsung, 208
saturated fats, 141
sciatica, 121
seasonal affective disorder (SAD), 188
seated spinal twist, 130–131
sedentary death syndrome, 100
self-actualization, 29
self-care, 27–28
    fatigue and, 37
    integration of beauty and wellness, 44–46, 48–49
    massage and, 173–177
    before providing client services, 51
    self-creation and, 219
self-esteem, 29
self-talk. *See* positive affirmation
sensory awareness, 167–169. *See also* aromatherapy; massage; music
    modulation, 80
    smell, 177–181
    sound, 76, 194–197, 202–204
    taste, 142, 158–161
    touch, 169–172
    vision, 184–193
shampoo bowls, 125
Shiatsu, 174
shoes, 124
shoulder stretches, 127
side stretch, 129
sight. *See* vision
Simon, David, 58–59
singing, 201
Sitali breath, 84–85
sixth sense, 168
skin care, 66, 75–76, 170
sleep, 66, 177
Slow Food Movement, 154
smell, sense of, 177–181. *See also* aromatherapy
smiling, 66
smudging, 63, 65
social needs, 28–29
Solar Plexus Chakra, 50, 192
Soul music, 199
sound, 76, 194. *See also* music
    listening skills and, 195
    for meditation, 202–203
    noise reduction products, 203–204
    vibrations, 195–197
sour taste, 159
spa. *See* salons

spirituality, 218
  beauty as, 41–43
  food and, 134–135, 155–158
  in salons, 61–64
  success and, 22
St. Agnes Hospital, 196
stress, 68–70. *See also* breathing
    exercises; meditation
  cortisol levels and, 44–45
  emotional, 77–79
  environmental, 72–76
  free radicals and, 71–72
  massage for, 173
  nutrition and, 162–163
  positive affirmation for, 77
  reducing, 65, 92–94, 103
  response to, 70–71
stretching exercises, 107, 126–132
success, 20–22
sugars, 145
sunlight, 119
Swedish massage, 174
sweet taste, 159
swimming, 108
synergy, 216–217

Tai Chi, 118
taste, sense of, 142, 158–161
teaching, 38
Teilhard de Chardin, Pierre, 219
tendinitis, 120
Third Eye Chakra, 50, 193
thoracic outlet syndrome, 121
Throat Chakra, 50, 193
thumbs, 123
Toffler, Alvin, 68
toning, 202
toxic smells, 179–180
toxic sound, 202–203
Trager Bodywork, 118
trance dance, 115–116
Twain, Mark, 100

Ujjayi breath, 86
University of Washington, 197
U.S. Department of Agriculture
    (USDA), 145, 149
U.S. National Institutes of Health, 53

varicose veins, 121
Vata dosha, 56–59. *See also* Ayurveda
Vedas, 88, 194, 221
vegetables, 151
veins, varicose, 121
ventilation, 76
vibrations, 195–197
vision, 184–188
  color and, 191–193
  eye care, 186–187
visualization. *See* creative visualization
vitamins, 71, 137
  antioxidants in, 146
  fat-soluble, 140–141
voice training, 201

walking, 108
water, 66, 141–143
weight-bearing exercise, 107, 108
Weil, Andrew, 189
Weiner, Edie, 68
Wellness Councils of America, 70, 76
wellness quotient, 47–48
white noise. *See* anti-noise technology
whole foods, 136–137. *See also*
    nutrition; organic plants
Willet, Walter, 149
Winter, Ruth, 75
Wolverton, B.C., 75
work-station equipment, 124–125
World Health Organization, 53, 70
World Wide Web, 218–220
wrists, 123, 129

yoga, 48–49, 91
  benefits of, 110
  resources for, 114
  stretches, 107, 126–132
Yoga: Mastering the Basics (Anderson
    and Sovik), 91
Yoga International, 114
Yoga Journal, 114
youthing practices, 65–66

Zone principle, 143